Plain English for Doctors
and Other Medical Scientists

Plain English for Doctors
and Other Medical Scientists

OSCAR LINARES, MD

DAVID DALY

GERTRUDE DALY

TO David with All My Love ♡

Gertrude Daly

OXFORD
UNIVERSITY PRESS

Oxford University Press is a department of the University of Oxford. It furthers the University's objective of excellence in research, scholarship, and education by publishing worldwide. Oxford is a registered trade mark of Oxford University Press in the UK and certain other countries.

Published in the United States of America by Oxford University Press
198 Madison Avenue, New York, NY 10016, United States of America.

Library of Congress Cataloging-in-Publication Data
Names: Linares, Oscar, 1957– author. | Daly, David, 1959– author. |
Daly, Gertrude, 1993– author.
Title: Plain English for doctors and other medical scientists / Oscar Linares, David Daly, Gertrude Daly.
Description: New York, NY : Oxford University Press, [2017] | Includes bibliographical references.
Identifiers: LCCN 2016041847 | ISBN 9780190654849 (pbk.)
Subjects: | MESH: Medical Writing
Classification: LCC R119 | NLM WZ 345 | DDC 808.06/661—dc23
LC record available at https://lccn.loc.gov/2016041847

This material is not intended to be, and should not be considered, a substitute for medical or other professional advice. Treatment for the conditions described in this material is highly dependent on the individual circumstances. And, while this material is designed to offer accurate information with respect to the subject matter covered and to be current as of the time it was written, research and knowledge about medical and health issues is constantly evolving and dose schedules for medications are being revised continually, with new side effects recognized and accounted for regularly. Readers must therefore always check the product information and clinical procedures with the most up-to-date published product information and data sheets provided by the manufacturers and the most recent codes of conduct and safety regulation. The publisher and the authors make no representations or warranties to readers, express or implied, as to the accuracy or completeness of this material. Without limiting the foregoing, the publisher and the authors make no representations or warranties as to the accuracy or efficacy of the drug dosages mentioned in the material. The authors and the publisher do not accept, and expressly disclaim, any responsibility for any liability, loss or risk that may be claimed or incurred as a consequence of the use and/ or application of any of the contents of this material.

9 8 7 6 5 4 3 2 1
Printed by Webcom Inc., Canada

We dedicate this book to the doctors and other medical scientists who write. They strive to make the world a better place by writing about new ways to understand, prevent, treat and cure disease.

CONTENTS

CONCEPT 3   **PRESENT LOGICAL REASONING CLEARLY**

PREFACE

Medicus incomprehensibilis is a condition that affects doctors and other medical scientists, causing them to write dull, lifeless prose that is hard to understand. In this book, we identify two causes: necessary scientific complexity and needless grammatical complexity. We show how to diagnose and treat *medicus incomprehensibilis*. This involves cutting needless grammatical complexity, using proven plain-English writing tips, while keeping essential scientific content.

Medicus incomprehensibilis wastes time for every reader, reduces understanding, and slows the spread of new medical knowledge. This prevents medical discoveries from reaching the widest reasonable audience. The widest reasonable audience includes anybody with an interest in the science, including people from other countries, and people in other specialties, sub-specialties, disciplines, or levels of training. Treating *medicus incomprehensibilis* saves time for every reader and improves understanding, thus speeding the spread of new medical knowledge.

This matters in the 21st century, when English is the global language of science. English-language medical journals contain discoveries from doctors and other medical scientists from around the world. Yet three out of four English users are not native speakers. Thus, it makes sense to write about complex science without using complex grammar.

This book is intended for doctors and other medical scientists who write for medical science journals, and anyone who aspires to do so. It is designed for classroom use, self-study and reference. While we focus on writing for medical science journals, most tips also apply to other medical or science writing situations.

Who are we and how did we come to write this book?

I, Oscar, am a doctor. My parents fled Cuba when I was three years old. I grew up in Miami speaking Spanish at home and English in school. I studied medicine in Spanish in the Dominican Republic and earned my medical degree there.

After finishing medical school, I came back to the United States for residency. Since I'd studied abroad, I had to take a test to qualify to work as a medical resident. Even though I knew the concepts, learning medical English was a big challenge. Luckily, both Spanish and English tend to use the same Latin and Greek medical terms, which made things easier.

I did my fellowship in geriatric medicine at the University of Michigan, and continued there for another 15 years as a visiting scholar. It was there I learned medical writing through years of research and working with other doctors and medical scientists.

Nobody ever actually taught me how to write about medicine. Instead, my advisors told me to read articles in the journal you want to write for, study their style, and imitate it. It was understood: You're joining an exclusive club. You've got to learn to write like members of the club.

This was hard advice to follow. Even after three years of training in internal medicine, I had a tough time reading articles in geriatric neuroscience. They used lots of long, formal sentences and impressive-sounding words. Many sentences were in passive voice. Before I could understand an article, I had to study it carefully with Stedman's Medical Dictionary at my side.

Whenever we wrote a scientific article, the writing process worked like this. The lead author does the first draft, distributes it to co-authors for review, and makes revisions. The senior author approves the final draft.

I always felt medical writing wasn't as clear as it could be. It certainly wasn't reaching a wide audience. Only about 100 people in the world could understand the articles we wrote. In fact, most of the best minds in medicine couldn't understand. A friend suggested I read Strunk and White's book, *The Elements of Style*. But, in those days, nobody in medicine seemed to know or care about writing in plain English.

It was only when I started working with David a few years ago that I started to see a better way to write. Together, we began to define *medicus incomprehensibilis*, describe its symptoms, and explain how to treat it.

I, David, am a lawyer. I learned about plain English over the years from books, people and lots of practice. I read Strunk and White's *The Elements of Style* in college. But nobody ever told me the ideas in that book might apply to math or music, my two college majors.

While studying in Germany during my junior year, I learned what it was like to be a "foreigner." While I and the other foreign students were among the best and brightest in every class, we always sat in the front row, straining to hear the professor clearly. We often had minor troubles understanding ideas written in a polite or formal German that differed from the German we spoke in everyday life.

In law school at the University of Michigan, I took the standard course on legal research and writing, where we read Wydick's book, *Plain English for Lawyers*. I organized weekly German and Spanish conversation tables at the dining hall. During my senior year, I taught the *Introduction to American Law* course for foreign legal scholars, which involved research and writing. These experiences helped me see some of the difficulties non-natives face in reading and writing English.

Years later, I found myself at Chrysler working on international business deals. There, I encountered many smart people, Americans and foreigners, who found traditional contract language hard to understand.

Like most lawyers, I had learned traditional legal writing by imitating other lawyers. When writing expert Bryan Garner came to Chrysler to put on seminars on plain English for the legal staff, I was skeptical. But I tried his ideas and found they worked. When he came back the next year, he pointed out my writing sample as one written in almost perfect plain English. Somewhere along the way, I also learned about Flesch Reading Ease scores. I found plain English was ideal for international automotive deals, where people in different disciplines from all over the world work together to build and sell cars.

After I had experience writing contracts in plain English, I wrote a few articles for the *Michigan Bar Journal*. One called, "Why Bother to Write Contracts in Plain English?"[i] has been cited on legal writing websites around the world. Another, "Taming the Contract Clause from Hell: A Case Study,"[ii] got criticized by a reader who thought my translation wasn't quite right. In my response article, "The Return of the Contract Clause from Hell,"[iii] I said he was right to call it a *"translation."* The original was so convoluted, it might as well have been written in a foreign language. Anything that bad was bound to be misunderstood. This whole exchange became the subject of Prof. Joseph Kimble's article, "The Great Myth that Plain Language is not Precise,"[iv] and a chapter in his book, *Lifting the Fog of Legalese: Essays on Plain Language.*[v]

We, Oscar and David, got the idea for this book a few years ago, when we started working together to revise a paper on some of Oscar's medical research. At first, we had a clash in writing styles. But after dozens of shouting matches, we worked everything out and the article got published. (One reviewer tried to turn our plain-English into traditional medical writing.)

The final draft was far better than the original, and we traced the improvement to a dozen or so principles. We thought other medical authors might benefit if we could explain them. We started by writing down a list of rules for plain English medical writing. One rule was, *Decide what you need to say, then say it clearly and concisely.*[vi] This general rule applies all the time. Other rules were specific (e.g., *talk in terms of one doctor treating one patient*), but only apply *usually, often,* or *sometimes.* Therefore, we thought it better to call these ideas, *tips.*

As we prepared to write, we checked other books on writing, found other tips, and added them to our list. A few books we particularly liked were Anne E. Greene's *Writing Science in Plain English*[vii] and Joseph Williams' *Style: Toward Clarity and Grace.*[viii] As we added other people's ideas to our own list of tips, we noticed some ideas were more general and some, more specific. Sometimes, different tips approached the same problem from a different angle. Some were numerical *(Keep the subject and verb together in the first seven or eight words)*, others grammatical or linguistic *(Prefer the short word)*, some conceptual *(Put the main point first)*. We decided to include some of these different approaches, since some readers might respond better to one approach or another.

I, Gertrude, graduated from the University of Michigan with a degree in English. I am now a writer and editor. I run a blog about royal families with about 75% of my followers outside the USA.

Like Oscar and David, I've also had experience studying in another country. During high school, I was an exchange student in Latvia. Some of my Latvian classmates spoke English better than others, but it always came out as a *Latvian* kind of English. They were obviously thinking in Latvian and translating their thoughts. They tended to use shorter sentences, simpler grammar, and particular words and phrases that translated well from Latvian into English. As they did this, I found myself talking more like them so we could communicate better.

Later on, when I studied medieval, renaissance and early-modern literature at the University of Michigan, I learned how English has changed over time. Jane Austin, Shakespeare, Chaucer and Beowulf: the further back you go, the harder it is for a modern audience to understand. I also learned how English has changed as it has spread throughout the world. In this book, we urge authors to write modern English, keeping essential scientific terms, which help explain the science, but without archaic, exotic or obscure language that might keep some readers from understanding.

How we structured the book

We grouped our plain-English writing tips into nine chapters. Each chapter covers a handful of related tips. We grouped these chapters into three concepts: reading ease, vivid language, and flow of logic.

The first concept, *Take charge of your reading ease score,* deals with objective measures of readability: the Flesch Reading Ease score and the Flesch-Kincaid Grade Level. We use these scores the way a doctor uses a blood pressure cuff, to quickly and easily get some useful information. Any good writer should know about these scores and how to use them to help improve their writing.

The second concept, *Prefer vivid language,* asks the reader to ponder the difference between the real world (e.g., *flesh and blood, bed pans, IV bags*) and the world of abstract ideas (e.g., *diagnoses, theories, concepts*). When you write, you should never leave your reader in doubt as to which world you're talking about.

The third concept is *Present logical reasoning clearly.* Logical flow is often good for a medical journal article. But sometimes, when you fix reading ease and use more vivid language, hidden problems with the flow of logic come to light. Once you can see the problem clearly, it's often easy to fix.

Another common problem is, sometimes an expert, an *insider* in their field, skips steps of logical reasoning that seem *"obvious"* to them. Their peer reviewers, also experts and insiders in their field, fail to notice the missing steps. But what is obvious to insiders may not be obvious to everybody else in the widest reasonable audience. Often, outsiders interested in the topic could follow the train of thought if only the expert would take care to spell out their steps of reasoning.

The tips in this book come with exercises, so you can practice what you learn. We base most exercises on excerpts from six leading medical journals: *Journal of the American Medical Association, The Lancet, New England Journal of Medicine, British Medical Journal, Mayo Clinic Proceedings,* and *American Family Physician.* We chose these journals since they represent today's best "standard" medical writing.

Writing in plain English is a skill you must hone by practice. Our goal is to point you in the right direction, give some general guidance and specific tips, and then, encourage you to develop your own creativity and good judgment. For most exercises, we conclude by asking you to *make any other changes you can think of to improve reading ease.*

For the exercises in Chapters 1–6, we check reading ease scores for the original excerpts and our revisions in the Exercise Key. In Chapter 7, we analyze these data to show how reading ease improves.

The tips in this book are specific, easy to use, and they really work. Many are simple (e.g., *Use normal sentence length*). Yet for each tip, we found examples in journals where the authors did the opposite, and the editors and peer reviewers let it pass.

Medical science writing is important. It is every medical writer's duty to write clearly and concisely. Learning to express complex ideas clearly and concisely is in no way a remedial skill. Rather, it can only been seen as a sign of mastery.

Notes

  i. Daly D, "Why Bother to Write Contracts in Plain English?" *Mich Bar J,* (August 1999): 850–851.
 ii. Daly D, "Taming the Contract Clause from Hell: a Case Study," *Mich Bar J,* (October 1999): 1155–1157.
iii. Daly D, "The Return of the Contract Clause from Hell," *Mich Bar J,* (February 2000): 202–204.
 iv. Kimble J, "The Great Myth That Plain Language Is Not Precise," *Scribes J Leg Writing* 7 (1998–2000), 109.
  v. Kimble J, *Lifting the Fog of Legalese: Essays on Plain Language* (Durham, NC: Carolina Academic Press, 2006): 37–48.
 vi. This rule came from one of Bryan Garner's live seminars.
vii. Greene A, *Writing Science in Plain English,* (Chicago: University of Chicago Press, 2013).
viii. Williams J, *Style: Lessons in Clarity and Grace,* 9th ed. (New York: Pearson Longman, 2007).

ACKNOWLEDGMENTS

We thank and acknowledge several people for their contributions:

For their years of mentorship and collaboration in writing about medical science and mathematical modeling: Raymond C. Boston, MSc, PhD, Abramson Cancer Center of the School of Medicine, Professor Emeritus of Biostatistics, Department of Biostatistics and Epidemiology, Perelman School of Medicine, University of Pennsylvania; William E. Schiesser, PhD, ScD, Emeritus McCann Professor of Chemical and Biomolecular Engineering and Professor of Mathematics at Lehigh University; Jeffrey B. Halter MD, Professor of Internal Medicine and Director, Geriatrics Center at the University of Michigan; and Loren A. Zech, MD, Senior Scientist, National Institutes of Health.

Bryan A. Garner for his live seminars on plain English writing at Chrysler Corporation and his many fine books on plain English.

Joseph Kimble, distinguished professor Emeritus, Western Michigan University—Cooley Law School, for his guidance and encouragement as editor of the plain English column of *The Michigan Bar Journal*, and as President of Clarity International.

Anne E. Greene for her book, *Writing Science in Plain English*, which in many ways served as a model for this book.

Miriam S. Daly, MD and Mary Laur for their review and comments on early drafts.

Janice L. Bernick, PhD, FNP; John J. Bernick, MD, PhD; William E. Maxwell, Jr., JD; and Annemarie L. Daly, MD, JD, FACP for their support and encouragement during the time we wrote this book.

Andrea Knobloch, Allison Pratt, Emily Perry, Cheryl Jung, Christopher Reid, Lani Oshima, and the other wonderful editors and staff at Oxford University Press who helped bring this book to print.

Introduction

Since writing is the only means the medical profession has of universally disseminating knowledge concerning new therapeutic concepts, medical discoveries, or clinical experience, it is the moral obligation of every physician who has made an original scientific observation or has formulated from his own experience a new medical theory, to publish it for the information of his colleagues, and the ultimate benefit of mankind. —Selma DeBakey[1]

A. Why bother to write in plain English?

Good writing takes work. If your article is good enough to get published, why should you make an extra effort to ensure it is clear, concise and readable? Here are ten reasons.

1. IT HELPS SPREAD NEW MEDICAL KNOWLEDGE

When doctors share ideas about theory and practice, it helps spread medical knowledge. New medical discoveries prevent illness, relieve suffering, find cures, and extend life. Difficult-to-understand writing slows down this process; clear, concise writing speeds it up.

2. IT HELPS TEACH THE PROFESSION

The Hippocratic Oath is a tradition of the medical profession; many doctors take it when they graduate from medical school. As part of the oath, they pledge to teach others the profession *"according to their ability and judgment."* This implies they'll do what they can to make medicine understandable to others.

3. IT SHOWS RESPECT FOR THE READER

Doctors are busy professionals. When you write in plain English, it shows respect. Your reader will read faster, understand better, and remember longer. Research in other fields shows 80% of readers prefer plain English.[2] Even if they can under-stand an article written in a traditional style, doctors are human too. Their brains work the same way as everybody else's. The same factors that influence reading ease for everybody else also influence reading ease for doctors.

4. IT SAVES READING TIME

How much time does the average doctor spend reading medical journals? Research published in the *Journal of the Medical Library Association* reports the average pediatrician spends 118 hours a year.[3] The *Journal of General Internal Medicine* reports the average internist spends 228 hours a year.[4]

What is the potential savings in reading time? Since there is little research on plain English medical writing, we can only make an educated guess based on experience in other fields. Writing expert Robert Eagleston thinks writing in plain English may cut reading time by 30% to 50%.[5] Joseph Kimble tested traditional and plain English contracts on various groups of readers and found that plain English cut reading time between 4.7% and 19.7% while improving comprehension.[6] Considering how much doctors read and how much time plain English saves, it seems likely that, if all medical journals were written in plain English, it could save the average doctor a week or two per year.

Writing well may take extra work, but even if it does, it's worth it. If your article is published and circulated to thousands of readers, any extra time you spend to write more clearly and concisely is small compared to the total time you save for your readers.

5. IT HELPS YOUR WORK REACH THE WIDEST REASONABLE AUDIENCE

When you consider the *widest reasonable audience*, and write in a style suitable for them, it promotes free and efficient exchange of new medical knowledge. Ideally, a medical journal article should be accessible to anybody interested in the subject matter, whether or not they are an *insider* in a field. This may include a doctor or scientist working in the same or a related specialty, a student, or a nurse. It includes regular journal subscribers and those who search for articles on the internet.

English is the global language of science, but many people who read English-language medical journals are not native speakers. In fact, according to English-language expert David Chrystal, non-native English speakers outnumber native speakers 3:1.[7] The widest reasonable audience includes those living or educated in an English-speaking country or elsewhere, whether a native speaker of English or not.

In Appendix 1, we present a survey of English speakers around the world. Some of the conclusions we reached in putting it together surprised us. For example, did you know there are now 23 countries where more than 10 million people speak English? Did you know there are more people who speak English in Asia than in North America? And did you know Germany is now the seventh largest English-speaking country in the world with more than 50 million English speakers? Many German doctors read English-language medical journals. They may have a first-rate medical education but only read English at a USA high school level. Given that English-language medical journals are read by doctors throughout the world, it makes good sense to write complex science in plain English.

6. IT HELPS PLEAD FOR A CAUSE

Medical science articles advocate for people who are poor, sick or oppressed. If you don't make your point clearly, you're not helping anybody. Writing in an inflated formal style sends the message *there's no urgent problem. It's just business as usual for those of us who work in a hospital, university or research center.* Writing in plain English helps send the message that a problem is important and urgent.

7. IT HELPS HUMANIZE YOUR WRITING

Writing in plain English sounds more natural, closer to the way people speak in everyday life. It sounds professional, with careful attention to the science, but less formal and bureaucratic. This means your writing sounds more human and puts less of a burden on your reader.

8. IT SHOWS RESPECT FOR YOUR WORK

Your research and ideas deserve to be presented clearly and concisely. Good writing helps build your reputation and benefits your career. More people will read your work and want to work with you.

9. IT HELPS OVERCOME EDITORIAL BLINDNESS

Writing in plain English helps you overcome *editorial blindness*, that feeling you get when you work on an article so long you miss problems a reader with a fresh eye would see. The tips in this book help you look at your writing from a fresh perspective.

10. IT SAVES TIME AND IMPROVES CONTENT

As a medical researcher, your time is valuable. Learning to write and revise in plain English may take some extra time and effort initially; but, once you learn how, it saves time for everybody. So ultimately, there is no extra cost.

Most medical journal articles involve multiple authors and go through peer review. This involves many people and many steps. Getting the first step right, by making sure your draft is clear and concise, saves time and effort at each later step.

Let's look at the process from the lead author's point of view. You start by writing the first draft as clearly and concisely as you can. Next, your co-authors review the draft. Since the draft is clear and concise, they focus more on content and less on form. They read faster, understand better, and give better comments. They become more personally invested in the work, and team morale improves.

Once you get comments, you incorporate them into a revised draft. Since the original was clear and concise, this revision goes quickly. Since you got better comments from your co-authors, the content gets better. Since you continue to check reading ease as you revise, the revised draft becomes even clearer and more concise.

Now, your co-authors review the second draft, which reflects everybody's comments. They see the improved content and this lifts team morale further. They become more invested in the research effort. You and your co-authors continue to review and revise as long as you need.

Once you're satisfied with the article, you submit it to a journal. If the journal likes it, they assign it for editorial and peer review. Just as with co-author review, this review goes faster and generates better comments.

Writing a first draft in plain English may take longer, but, after that, each step of review and revising goes faster and helps improve clarity, conciseness and content. As a result, you end up with a better paper, possibly with no more time and effort.

You can't learn to write in plain English just by reading a book. You must put your own pen to paper.[8] This is why we included exercises for each chapter.

Exercise A. Widest reasonable audience
Look at Appendix 2, Excerpt 1 from *Mathematical Modeling of Kidney Transport: Glomerular Filtration.*

1. What types of people might want to read an article about modeling how a kidney filters blood? In other words, who is the widest reasonable audience?
2. What changes would you suggest to make the article clearer for different people in the widest reasonable audience? (E.g., a mathematician might need a better explanation about kidney anatomy.)

Compare your answers to the Exercise Key in Appendix 3.

B. What do we mean by *plain English*?

When we talk about plain English, we mean writing that conveys the right content, clearly and concisely. Some people think writing in plain English involves dumbing down medical science, but this is not so. Rather, it involves sharpening up the science to make it clearer and more accessible to the widest reasonable audience.

By *content*, we mean *essential scientific content*, those important scientific ideas an author must include in their article. What content is non-essential? Sometimes, an author loads down a sentence with asides and parentheticals that only loosely relate to the main idea. Only an author can judge what content is, or isn't, essential. An author should never sacrifice essential content to make their article easy to read, but they might cut non-essential content.

Writing is *clear* when the narrative uses words and concepts familiar to the reader. Ideally, a reader can understand and vividly imagine the article on first reading without having to *study* it. The reader remembers each key idea.

Writing is *concise* when it demands as little of the reader's mental energy as possible. This usually means short while still clear. Good writing involves trade-offs. A few short words may convey the message more vividly than one long but lifeless word. Writing concisely means cutting an unnecessary word, but cutting too many words may make the message cryptic and harder to understand. For example, a math equation is very concise, but a reader might understand the same idea better if the author explained it in words first.

Figure I-1 presents a diagram that shows how we think about plain English. Within the universe of all the possible ways you might write a medical journal article, plain English represents the intersection of three ideas: (1) essential scientific content (2) presented clearly and (3) concisely. This diagram represents plain English—*what* we are trying to achieve. We devote the rest of this book to explaining *how* to achieve it.

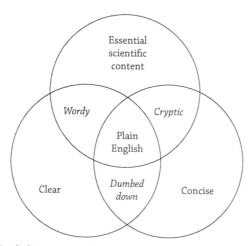

Figure I-1 Plain English is essential scientific content, presented clearly and concisely.

Exercise B. How does sentence length affect reading ease?
Appendix 2 contains excerpts from three articles from medical science journals.
Read the first paragraph of each out loud.

1. Count the number of words in each sentence and compute the average sentence length. Which excerpt uses the longest sentences? The shortest?
2. Which excerpt do you find easiest to read? The hardest?
3. Judging from these excerpts, do you see any link between reading ease and sentence length?

Compare your answers to the Exercise Key in Appendix 3.

C. *Medicus incomprehensibilis*

Open any leading medical journal today and you'll find an article that shows symptoms of *medicus incomprehensibilis,* a condition that affects doctors and other medical scientists, causing them to write dull, lifeless prose that is hard to understand. *Medicus incomprehensibilis* wastes time for every reader. It conveys the scientific message less clearly, vividly and memorably. It keeps some readers from fully understanding. It causes others to give up, since reading becomes too tedious. It excludes any potential reader who might understand the science, but can't deal with the complex writing style.

Can we explain *medicus incomprehensibilis* just by the inherent complexity of medical science? No. Certainly, in order to understand a medical journal article, a reader must know something about biology, chemistry, physics, anatomy, epidemiology, pharmacology, mathematics and statistics. But in many cases, complex science is a distant secondary cause of *medicus incomprehensibilis.* The primary cause is a needlessly complex traditional medical writing style, which overuses several writing habits. See Table I-1. Any one of these symptoms is not necessarily

Table I-1. **Symptoms of *medicus incomprehensibilis*: over-used writing habits**

Low reading ease	*Abstraction*	*Unclear logical reasoning*
• long sentence (>25 words)	• abstract language	• long paragraph
• run-on sentence	• formality	• awkwardly organized
• dependent clause	• nominalization	information
• parenthetical statement	• plural subject	• unclear paragraph topic
• long word	• obscure jargon	• unclear narrative pathway
• unnecessary word ending		• missing step of logical
• noun string		reasoning
• passive voice		

Table I-2. **Exercise C. Symptoms of *medicus incomprehensibilis* observed**

	Excerpt 1	*Excerpt 2*	*Excerpt 3*
Low reading ease	✓	✓	✓
long sentence (>25 words)			
run-on sentence			
dependent clause			
parenthetical statement			
long word			
passive voice			
Abstraction	✓	✓	✓
abstract language			
nominalization			
formality			
plural subjects			
obscure jargon			

a problem. But the more symptoms a piece of writing has, the worse the case of *medicus incomprehensibilis*.

Exercise C. Recognizing symptoms of medicus incomprehensibilis
Look again at the excerpts from the three journal articles in Appendix 2. Read the first paragraph or two of each and make a checkmark in Table I-2 to indicate each symptom of *medicus incomprehensibilis* you observe.

Compare your answers to the Exercise Key in Appendix 3.

D. Using the tips in your writing

The tips in this book can serve as a checklist to help you write and revise more efficiently. For example, if you take care to follow the tip, *Use normal sentence length*, you will never waste time writing and revising a 50-word sentence. If you read the tips and do the exercises, you will learn how to write medical science in plain English. As you apply the tips, your writing will start to improve right away. With steady practice, it will continue to improve.

"TIPS"—NOT RULES

Everybody who writes a book about writing style gives a list of rules. In developing our list, we checked other books and articles and tried to include all the best ideas that apply to medical writing. (See Resources.)

Like medicine, writing is both an art and a science. It involves many choices about how to say things. There is only one *rule* for plain English medical writing: *Decide what you need to say, then say it clearly and concisely.* This rule applies all the time.

We call the other suggestions in this book *tips*. Most are specific and easy to apply. We expect an author to use good judgment about when a tip may prove helpful. We offer each tip with the provisos: "when it helps," "when it works," "when it makes sense," and "if it isn't confusing, distracting, or vulgar." For example, one tip is, *Prefer active voice.* Many medical writers use passive voice too much and their reading ease and vividness suffer as a result. But, if you use passive voice sparingly, it can work well.

Think of each tip like a tool in your toolbox of writing skills. Like any tool, not every tip helps in every situation. A hammer doesn't help much to fix a clogged sink. If a tool doesn't work in a particular situation, that doesn't mean you throw it away. Instead, you keep it in your toolbox for when it serves a useful purpose.

PLAIN ENGLISH WRITING TIPS HELP IMPROVE ALL KINDS OF WRITING

Many medical journal articles suffer from *medicus incomprehensibilis*; some are worse than others. Some are almost unreadable. Some are tedious. Some are readable, but take study. Still others are easy to read, but wordy. In this book, we address each of these issues. The tips we provide can help make *poor* writing *good*, and *good* writing *better*. Don't stop improving just because you feel your writing is *good enough*.

SMALL CHANGES ADD UP

Some of the writing tips we present in this book may seem trivial, but many small changes quickly add up to a big improvement in reading ease and clarity. Each individual tip may only improve your article's reading ease score by a few points, make one idea a little more vivid, or improve the flow of logic in a small way. But by making many small changes, you may see your reading ease score jump, a hazy idea become clear, or a weak chain of logical reasoning become strong.

KAIZEN (改善)

Japanese quality management principles used in industry have strongly influenced our way of writing about medicine. Kaizen, the Japanese term for *improvement* or *self-changing for the best of all*, refers to a philosophy and a set of practices that focus upon improving any process. By improving processes, kaizen aims to eliminate waste. Kaizen is a daily process, which goes beyond improving productivity. It is also a process that, when done correctly, humanizes the workplace, eliminates overly hard work (*muri*), and teaches people how to spot and eliminate waste in business processes. While kaizen usually delivers small improvements, the culture of continual small improvements yields large productivity improvements.[9]

CHALLENGING CONVENTION

Some of our tips differ from traditional notions about "proper" medical writing. We challenge any convention that serves no scientific purpose, yet makes an article needlessly complex or abstract. If you ever feel one of our tips violates a convention of the profession, ask yourself, *Is this convention based on a scientific reason, or a social reason?* If the reason is *scientific*, by all means, follow the convention.

But if the convention is based on a *social* reason, ask yourself, *How important is that social reason? Is it more important than respecting a reader's time? Is it more important than making an idea accessible to the widest reasonable audience?* The benefits of plain-English outweigh any superficial notion about "proper" writing.

You might ask, *Aren't medical writing habits that contribute to medicus incomprehensibilis of long standing?* Not so much as some people think. Many medical writers of the past wrote their scientific works clearly. For example, Edward Jenner's 1798 paper, "An Inquiry into the Causes and Effects of the Variolae Vacciniae, or Cow-Pox," which first coined the term *vaccination,*[10] was written for a wide audience and does not overuse difficult scientific language. Watson and Crick's 1953 article, "Molecular Structure of Nucleic Acids: A Structure for Deoxyribose Nucleic Acid," which first proposed the double-helix structure of DNA, is short and readable.[11]

STAGES OF GRIEF

If you've spent years learning to write in the traditional medical writing style, you may feel a deep sense of grief and loss in reading this book, since it reveals weaknesses of the traditional style. If so, you may go through some of the stages of grief Elisabeth Kübler-Ross described in her book, *On Death and Dying.* These stages of grief are *denial, anger, bargaining, depression,* and *acceptance.*[12] We worked through some of these same feelings in planning and writing this book.

If you never learned to write in the traditional medical style, so much the better. We hope this book spares you any such feelings of grief and loss, but we also urge you to be patient with those who are going through the grieving process.

E. Notes on the exercises

Anybody who wants to learn to prevent, diagnose and treat *medicus incomprehensibilis* must spend some time revising writing samples. The exercises give you a chance to practice applying the tips to excerpts from published journal articles. We give our own revisions in the Exercise Key in Appendix 3.

You may feel uneasy trying to rewrite somebody else's work. Like dissecting a cadaver, this may seem unpleasant, but it is a part of learning.

Don't worry if your revision differs from ours. Each revision reflects our understanding of the excerpt taken out of context. We had two MD's review each exercise. But in some cases, we weren't sure what the original was trying to say, even after careful study. We don't claim our revision is the best possible, or that it's better than the original.

Don't interpret the fact we chose any excerpt as criticism. In some cases, we just wanted a sample of medical writing for you to practice on.

Most exercises focus on one tip, but also ask you to make any other changes you can think of to improve reading ease. This is how revising works: you set out to fix one thing, and as you do, you see other things to fix. Our revisions reflect applying many tips, not just the one featured in the exercise.

Somebody might say one of our revisions isn't entirely correct, changes the meaning or sense of the original, over-simplifies something, or loses some essential scientific content. Despite our best efforts, we know this may be so. If a revision doesn't involve the author, it's hard to be sure whether it is correct or captures the sense of the original. If we made any mistake, or if anybody interprets a passage in a different way, perhaps the original wasn't clear. In any event, losing key content is never a problem for an author revising their own work. Our goal is to teach you to revise your own work, not to *translate* other people's work.

Conclusion

If you've read this far, you've already taken the biggest step toward writing better. You accept that it's possible to write about medicine in plain English and that it's worthwhile. Most importantly, you're willing to try.

Notes

1. DeBakey S, "Suggestions on Preparation of Medical Papers," *JAMA* 155, no. 18 (1954): 1573.
2. Kimble, *Lifting the Fog of*, 3–13 (see Preface, n. 5).
3. Tenopir C, et al. "Journal Reading Patterns and Preferences of Pediatricians," *J Med Libr Assoc* 95, no. 1 (2007), under "Background," http://www.ncbi.nlm.nih.gov/pmc/articles/PMC1773049/.
4. Saint S, et al. "Journal Reading Habits of Internists," *J Gen Intern Med* 15, no. 12 (December 2000), under "Reading Habits," http://www.ncbi.nlm.nih.gov/pmc/articles/PMC1495716/.

5. Collins L, "Plea for Plain English," *QNP* (December 9, 1993): 33.

6. Kimble J, "Answering the Critics of Plain Language," *Scribes Journal of Legal Writing* 5 (1994–1995): 70–71.

7. Crystal D, *English as a Global Language,* 2nd ed. (Cambridge: Cambridge University Press, 2003), 69.

8. Wydick R, *Plain English for Lawyers* (Durham, NC, Carolina Academic Press, 2005): 6.

9. *Wikipedia*, s.v. "Kaizen," https://en.wikipedia.org/wiki/Kaizen (accessed August 9, 2015).

10. Jenner E, "An Inquiry into the Causes and Effects of the Variolae Vacciniae, or Cow-Pox," in *The Harvard Classics*, ed. Charles W. Eliot (New York: Collier) 38: 153–180.

11. Watson J, Crick F, "Molecular Structure of Nucleic Acids: A Structure for Deoxyribose Nucleic Acid," *Nature* 171, no. 4356 (April 1953): 737–738.

12. Kübler-Ross E, *On Death and Dying* (New York: Scribner, 2003).

TAKE CHARGE OF YOUR READING EASE SCORE

Everything that can be thought at all can be thought clearly. Everything that can be said can be said clearly.—Ludwig Wittgenstein[1]

In the first three chapters, we discuss how you can improve your writing by improving your reading ease scores. We address reading ease first, since it represents the "low hanging fruit" of writing in plain English.

A. Flesch Reading Ease and Flesch-Kincaid Grade Level tests

Flesch Reading Ease is a readability test that indicates how difficult it is to read a passage in English. The scores generally range from 0.0 to 100.0. Higher scores indicate material that is easier to read; lower scores, more difficult. It's possible for a passage to have a negative score.[2]

The *Flesch–Kincaid Grade Level*, a related test, assigns a USA school grade level to a reading passage. Both tests were developed by the United States Navy as a way to assess how difficult a passage of text is to read. Both tests use the same core measures, word length and sentence length, but use different weight factors. The tests are objective, since they consider only form and not content.[3,4] The results of the two tests correlate roughly inversely. A text with a high reading ease score should have a low grade level score. Table C1-1 shows an approximate correlation of the reading ease and grade level scores.

A writing sample is generally considered to be in plain English if it falls in the 60–70 range for reading ease and has about an 8 or 9 grade level.[5] What scores

Table C1-1. **Flesch Reading Ease vs. Flesch-Kincaid Grade Level[1]**

Reading ease score	Grade level score
90 to 100	5th grade
80 to 90	6th grade
70 to 80	7th grade
60 to 70	8th and 9th grade
50 to 60	10th to 12th grade (high school)
30 to 50	college/university (13 to 16)
0 to 30	college/university graduate (17 and above)

[1]Flesch, "How to Write in," (see Concept 1, n. 4).

should we expect for plain-English medical writing? Because medical writing uses Latin or Greek names and other scientific terms, we think a good reading ease score tends to be a bit lower (about 46–70), and the grade level a bit higher (about 7–11). We show in Chapter 7 how we came up with these ranges.[6]

WHY WORRY ABOUT READING EASE?

The Flesch Reading Ease and Flesch–Kincaid Grade Level tests give a good general idea of how difficult it is to read a passage of text. They are also quick and easy to calculate. Chances are your computer's spell checker can calculate them for you.

We use these tests the way a doctor uses a blood pressure cuff, to get some useful information quickly at low cost. We often use them in a way that is "off label," to check just one sentence or paragraph rather than a whole article. But, the shorter the block of text, the more unreliable the score may be in reflecting actual reading ease. Some things are probably not so hard for a doctor to read as the score might suggest (e.g., names of body parts, medicines, surgical procedures).

WHERE CAN YOU FIND THESE TESTS?

The Flesch Reading Ease and Flesch-Kincaid Grade Level tests come as a standard feature of the MS Word spelling and grammar checker. They are also bundled with other popular word processing programs and services. (You may need to enable style checking on your word processing program. Check the program's website for user help.) Different versions may provide slightly different scores. If your word processing program doesn't have these tests, you can find them free online (https://readability-score.com).

SHIFTING THE CURVE FOR READING EASE SCORES

Journal articles written in a traditional medical writing style naturally have a range of reading ease scores. The scores for any individual article depend upon the article's science content and the author's writing style. We might draw a curve to represent the range of reading ease scores for different journal articles, something like Figure C1-1. (See left side—"Traditional.") Here, we represent the mean Flesch Reading Ease score for traditional medical writing as "μ_T."

By taking care to improve reading ease scores, it ought to be possible to shift the entire curve to the right. (See right side—"Plain English.") After this shift, the reading ease scores will still vary, depending upon each article's science content and the authors' writing style. We represent the mean reading ease score for plain English medical writing as "μ_{PE}."

B. WSEG scores—How we track key reading ease data

We find four items of data helpful to assess reading ease for a passage of text: the number of <u>w</u>ords (w), average <u>s</u>entence length (s), Flesch Reading <u>E</u>ase score (E), and Flesch-Kincaid <u>G</u>rade Level (G). We abbreviate these four items of information as "WSEG." For example, if a paragraph has 36 words, an average sentence length of 18.0 words, a reading ease score of 71.0, and a grade level of 7.8, we would summarize this information as *(WSEG = 36/18.0/71.0/7.8).* We use WSEG scores to track changes in reading ease throughout this book.

Example—Using reading ease scores to help diagnose and treat medicus incomprehensibilis

It is possible to detect symptoms of *medicus incomprehensibilis* even in garden-variety traditional medical writing. For example, here is a sentence from an

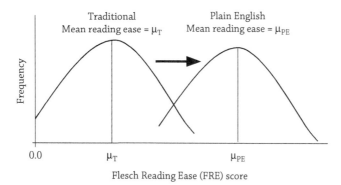

Figure C1-1 Plain English can materially improve a journal's reading ease.

article in the *American Family Physician,* a journal read by 190,000 family practice doctors.

> Referral to a clinical geneticist for assistance in the diagnosis and management of Noonan syndrome, including determining the appropriateness and sequence of genetic testing, may be helpful.[7] *(WSEG = 27/27.0/0.0/20.7)*

We understand this sentence, but it's not as easy to read as it might be. An occasional sentence like this doesn't pose a problem for the average medical journal reader. But when every sentence sounds like this, an article soon becomes tedious and fails to serve the widest reasonable audience.

The *WSEG* score gives us a few hints about this sentence. First, it is a little long: one sentence of 27 words. The reading ease score is 0.0. The grade level is 20.7, which may not pose a problem for a doctor educated in English. But it might for a doctor educated in another language.

What makes this sentence challenging to read—the science or the writing style? Certainly, understanding the term, *Noonan syndrome,* requires some medical knowledge. But, in this case, the whole article is about *Noonan syndrome;* the reader will likely learn what it involves. A reader can also tell *Noonan syndrome* is a medical condition. Thus, the science is a not the cause for this sentence's low reading ease.

As we see it, the low reading ease springs from commonly overused writing habits:

- Many words come between the subject *(referral)* and the verb *(may)*
- A long sentence—27 words
- A long dependent clause in the middle *(including determining the appropriateness and sequence of genetic counseling)*
- Abstract nouns: *referral, assistance, diagnosis, management, appropriateness* and *sequence*
- Slight redundancy—determining the *sequence* of genetic testing is part of determining *appropriateness*

If we try to revise the example to keep the same scientific content, but avoid or minimize these writing habits, we might end up with something like the revision in Table C1-2.

In this revision, the number of words is the same, but since the words are shorter, it takes up less space on the page. Since it uses two sentences, the average sentence length is one-half. The Flesch Reading Ease score jumps from 0.0 to 61.5. The grade level goes down from 20.7 to 8.0. Clearly, if every sentence

Table C1-2. **Revising to reduce *medicus incomprehensibilis***

	Original	Revised
Text	Referral to a clinical geneticist for assistance in the diagnosis and management of Noonan syndrome, including determining the appropriateness and sequence of genetic testing, may be helpful. (*WSEG* = 27/27/0.0/20.7)	It may help to refer a patient with Noonan syndrome to a clinical geneticist. They can help diagnose and manage it and help decide on genetic tests. (*WSEG* = 27/13.5/ 61.5/8.0)
Words	27	27
Average words per sentence	27	13.5
Reading ease score	0.0	61.5
Grade level	20.7	8.0

in every article could be revised like this, a journal could serve a much wider audience.

Is this the best possible revision? Maybe you can think of something better. Or maybe you would have made some different revising decisions than we did and achieved a different *WSEG* score. The point is, when you focus on reading ease, you can often make a big improvement.

Exercise D. Take charge of your reading ease score

1. Read the following excerpt out loud and underline each word with three syllables or more (but skip *expanded* and *produces*, which are two-syllable words that add common endings).
2. For each word you underlined, can you think of a shorter word or a few short words that mean close to the same thing? Or else, do you consider it an essential scientific term, not easy to replace?
3. Revise the excerpt to break up the long sentences into shorter ones. Keep any essential scientific term, but use shorter words where you can. Do you find your revision easier to read than the original?

Compare your answers to the Exercise Key in Appendix 3.

> **Given the complexity of the immune system, the development of an individual B cell is unlikely to follow a predictable and well-executed series of decision points whereby an antigen-reactive cell is expanded to a clone that produces a single antibody. A more realistic perspective is that their development depends on a series of error-prone, random rearrangement events and mutations whereby specificity for the original antigen is maintained (or not) by selective pressures.[8]**

Conclusion

The first concept is *Take charge of your reading ease score.* A reading ease score is based on two factors: average sentence length and average word length. In the next three chapters, we give tips for improving reading ease scores:

1. Use normal sentence length
2. Prefer the short word
3. Omit any needless word

Notes

1. Williams, *Style: Lessons in Clarity,* 3 (see Preface, n. 8).
2. For the exercises in this book, negative scores are truncated to zero. This is a standard feature for the MS word style checker. We present an analysis of the WSEG scores for excerpts used in Chapters 1–6 exercises and our revisions in Chapter 7. For this analysis, we calculated negative scores manually.
3. *Wikipedia,* s.v. "Flesch-Kincaid Readability Tests," https://en.wikipedia.org/wiki/Flesch%E2%80%93Kincaid_readability_tests (accessed February 14, 2016).
4. Flesch R, "How to Write in Plain English," *University of Canterbury,* http://www.mang.canterbury.ac.nz/writing_guide/writing/flesch.shtml (accessed February 12, 2016).
5. Ibid.
6. In general, these ranges represent one standard deviation around the mean of our model revisions. See our analysis in Chapter 7.
7. Bhambhani V, Muenke M, "Noonan Syndrome," *Am Fam Phys* 89, no. 1 (January 2014): 40.
8. Carter R, "B Cells in Health and Disease," *Mayo Clinic Proc* 81, no. 3 (March 2006), under "B Cells and Disease States," http://www.mayoclinicproceedings.org/article/S0025-6196(11)61466-3/fulltext.

CHAPTER 1

Use normal sentence length

Modern English, especially written English, is full of bad habits which spread by imitation and which can be avoided if one is willing to take the necessary trouble.—George Orwell, *Politics and the English Language*[1]

What makes traditional medical writing hard to read? One thing is long sentences. Controlling sentence length helps improve your reading ease score. Consider the following excerpt from Watson and Crick's 1953 article in *Nature*, which first described the double-helix structure of DNA:

> We wish to put forward a radically different structure for the salt of deoxyribose nucleic acid. This structure has two helical chains each coiled round the same axis (see diagram). We have made the usual chemical assumptions, namely, that each chain consists of phosphate di-ester groups joining β-D-deoxyribofuranose residues with 3', 5' linkages. The two chains (but not their bases) are related by a dyad perpendicular to the fibre axis. Both chains follow right-handed helices, but owing to the dyad, the sequences of the atoms in the two chains run in opposite directions. Each chain loosely resembles Furberg's model No. 1; that is, the bases are on the inside of the helix and the phosphates on the outside.[2]
>
> *(WSEG = 118/19.6/52.7/10.0)*

Even though this excerpt describes a complex topic in molecular biology, the average sentence length is less than 20 words. The reading ease score is 52.7 and the grade level is 10.0.

A. Keep sentence length 15 words average, 25 words maximum

Medical writing often needs to use long medical terms. Because of this, achieving a good reading ease score requires keeping the average sentence length under control. We think this means about 15 words average and 25 words maximum. Of course, when we say, *15 words average*, we mean some sentences are longer and some shorter.

There are exceptions. For example, you might write a longer sentence if your sentence ends in a list, or if you quote the long title of a study. Generally, if a sentence runs more than 25 words, it covers more than one idea and you should consider splitting it into two or more sentences. You'll find it's often easy to split up a long sentence to make shorter ones.

Writing style experts recommend mixing long and short sentences.[3] Many short sentences, one after another, can seem choppy and distract the reader. Many long sentences, one after another, become tedious to read.

NO SCIENTIFIC REASON FOR LONG SENTENCES

The science of reading ease tells us long sentences tend to be hard to read. In this respect, there is a good scientific reason to avoid long sentences. A complex idea may take longer to explain, but sentences of moderate length will serve just as well or better.

COMMON WISDOM ABOUT SENTENCE LENGTH MAY NOT APPLY TO MEDICAL WRITING

Experts in other fields recommend different "ideal" average sentence lengths ranging from 15 to 25 words.[4] Some writing experts actually teach techniques for writing long sentences.[5] This may do for fiction, which seeks to entertain, surprise and delight the readers and which tends to use fairly short words. However, studies show that, of all kinds of writing, fiction tends to use the shortest sentences.[6]

Trying to write longer sentences may work in other fields, but medical science writing calls for keeping average sentence length at the shorter end of range of "ideal" average sentence lengths.

There are several reasons why this is so. First, unlike fiction, medical writing seeks primarily to inform or persuade the reader and not to entertain. Second, medical writing uses long terms to describe diseases, medicines, chemicals and processes. These long terms tend to lower reading ease scores. An author should compensate for these scientific terms by avoiding needlessly long sentences.

Third, unlike most other fields (e.g., law and government regulation) medical writing reaches a global audience. Many, if not most, readers of medical science journals don't speak English as their first language. An article published in a major English-language journal will be read by doctors throughout the world. Even many doctors and medical scientists who work in English-speaking countries originally came from somewhere else.

Because of their unique subject matter, terms and audience, a medical author should strive for an average sentence length of about 15 words and a maximum sentence length of about 25 words.

Exercise 1. A. Keep sentence length 15 words average, 25 words maximum
For each sentence:

1. Read it out loud and count the number of words.
2. Revise to make shorter sentences. Make any other changes you can think of to improve reading ease.
3. Count the number of words for each new sentence and the total number of words. Compute the average number of words per sentence.

Compare your answers to the Exercise Key in Appendix 3.

1. But the physician's subsequent choice to designate the hospital discharge as against medical advice and pursue the formalized process associated with it (eg, specialized discharge forms) has no evidence-based utility for patient care, is not legally required, and has been shown to be associated with reduced willingness for the patient to return for future care.[7]

2. Our Review will focus on advances in understanding of COPD and its risk factors, prevalence, and natural history since these Reviews were published, address some of the questions that still persist, and raise some of the issues that health-care planners will have to consider as the burden of COPD increases as the world's population ages.[8]

3. Since *CYP2C9* explained 6 to 10 percent of the variability in these two patient samples, the *VKORC1* genotype appears to be the most important genetic factor determining variability in warfarin dose: in both clinical populations its effect was approximately three times that of the *CYP2C9* genotype.[9]

4. A systematic review of randomized clinical trials of multiple risk factor interventions for preventing ischaemic heart disease had a modest effect on changes in lifestyle factors, cholesterol concentrations, and blood pressure—the last two mainly owing to the drug treatment used—but no significant effect on long term mortality due to ischaemic heart disease.[10]

5. Over the past 100 years, the science of exercise has grown from seminal discoveries documenting the effects of exercise intensity on vascular control, heat production, oxygen requirement, and lactic acid dynamics—which led to Nobel Prizes in physiology or medicine in 1920 (August Krogh, Denmark) and 1922 (A.V. Hill, United Kingdom and Otto Meyerhof, Germany)—to our modern-day

understanding that one's cardiorespiratory fitness (indexed by one's maximum rate of oxygen consumption) is among the most powerful predictors of morbidity and mortality.[11]

6. In a prospective study in the Netherlands that followed more than 30,000 students 10 to 14 years of age for up to three years, annual scoliosis screening in addition to the usual biennial health checkup detected no cases of idiopathic scoliosis requiring surgery, and the authors concluded that additional annual scoliosis screening was not needed.[12]

B. Keep the subject and verb close together in the first seven or eight words

One thing that makes a sentence hard to read is having the subject and verb far apart. (See the Glossary if you need a refresher on the terms *subject* and *verb*.) This is especially true if the subject or verb is buried deep within a long sentence. Putting the subject and verb close together, near the start of the sentence, is a simple way to improve reading ease. This avoids the common problem of the reader losing track of the subject or verb and having to go back.[13,14]

Exercise 1.B. Keep the subject and verb close together in the first seven or eight words
For each sentence:

1. Read it out loud and underline the <u>subject once</u> and the <u>verb twice</u>. Count the number of words that come between them. Do the subject and verb come within the first eight words?
2. Revise to make new shorter sentences. Each new sentence should have its subject and verb close together within the first seven or eight words. Make any other changes you can think of to improve reading ease.

Compare your answers to the Exercise Key in Appendix 3.

1. Although SDM is well accepted in overtly value-laden clinical decisions such as prostate-specific antigen testing and mammography screening, the principles of SDM apply to a broad range of health care decisions, discharges against medical advice included.[15]

Note: *SDM* stands for *shared decision making.*

2. The only comprehensive effort to date to estimate summary measures of population health for the world, by cause, is the ongoing Global Burden of Diseases, Injuries, and Risk Factors (GBD) enterprise.[16]

3. Although drug effect is a complex phenotype that depends on many factors, early and often dramatic examples involving succinyl-choline and isoniazid facilitated acceptance of the fact that inheritance can have an important influence on the effect of a drug.[17]

4. Transparent reporting of review methods and detailed reporting of the clinical and methodological characteristics of the included studies and their results are important to enable a reader to judge the reliability of both the review and the individual studies and to assess their relevance to clinical practice and the meaning of the results reported in the review.[18]

5. Baseline demographic characteristics and the distribution of peri-operative ARDS risk factors or modifiers among those who did and did not develop postoperative ARDS (first procedure only) after bleo-mycin therapy are presented in table 2.[19]

Note: *ARDS* stands for *acute respiratory distress syndrome.*

6. Because patients often are reluctant to discuss traumatic events and may avoid treatment as a result, it is important to elicit patient preferences for treatment interventions.[20]

C. Put the main point first and then give commentary, detail or support

Sometimes, a sentence starts with a dependent clause that gives some commentary, detail or support before stating the main idea. This works well for a short sentence. For example:

> As with many autoimmune diseases, celiac disease is about two to three times more common in women.[21] (*WSEG=17/17.0/50.2/10.4*)

It also makes sense to state your premises before you state a conclusion.

But when a writer starts a long sentence with a long dependent clause, it can tax the reader's powers of concentration. For example, consider the sentence below where the main point starts 18 words into the sentence (in italics). We can improve reading ease by breaking up the long sentence, putting the main point first, and minimizing other long words (Table 1-1).

Sometimes a long sentence contains several key points. In such a case, it helps to split up a long sentence into shorter sentences, with each key point near the start of its own sentence.

If you want to help a busy reader understand your ideas, put the main point first, and then give commentary, detail or support.

Table 1-1. **Put the main point first**

Original	Revised
Although reducing heart rate will decrease myocardial oxygen consumption and will improve diastolic function and coronary perfusion, *for patients with sepsis, an inadequate chronotropic response may potentially negatively affect cardiac output and tissue perfusion.*[i] *(WSEG = 34/34.0/0.0/24.3)*	*For a patient with sepsis, a slow heart rate may cut cardiac output and tissue perfusion.* For a patient without sepsis, slowing the heart rate slows the heart's oxygen use. It also helps diastolic function and coronary perfusion. *(WSEG = 38/12.6/55.9/8.6)*

[i]Morelli A, et al. "Effect of Heart Rate Control with Esmolol on Hemodynamic and Clinical Outcomes in Patients with Septic Shock," *JAMA* 310, no. 16 (2013): 1689.

Exercise 1.C. Put the main point first and then give commentary, detail or support
For each sentence:

1. Read it out loud and underline the <u>main point</u> or each <u>key point</u>.
2. Count the number of words that come before the main point or each key point.
3. Does the main point come near the start of the sentence? If not, revise to break up any long sentence. Put the main point first or put each key point near the start of its own sentence. Make any other changes you can think of to improve reading ease.

Compare your answers to the Exercise Key in Appendix 3.

1. Although Ontario surgeons receive a premium and bill accurately when they operate urgently between 12 AM and 7 AM, the times and length of the overnight procedure and also how fatigued the surgeon truly was when starting elective cases the next day were unknown.[22]

2. First, estimates for 2000 of under-5 mortality, measured as the probability of death between 0 years and 5 years of age ($_5q_0$), and mortality as a young adult or middle-aged adult, measured as the probability of death between 15 years and 60 years of age ($_{45}q_{15}$),[23] were developed after review of available vital registration, sample registration, and census data and the application of the synthetic extinct generation and growth balance methods to correct for under-registration of deaths.[24]

3. The trial showed that pharmacogenetic-guided initiation of warfarin therapy resulted in a greater percentage of time in the therapeutic range, fewer excessive INRs, a shorter median time to therapeutic INR, and fewer dose adjustments.[25]

Note: *INR* stands for *international normalized ratio.*

4. The participation rate was lower than we expected when we did the power calculations; however, taking into account the fact that more people than expected had an increased risk and received counselling and that not even a trend to a reduction in ischaemic heart disease was observed, we doubt that a participation rate of 70% would have made any difference.[26]

5. Recommended CRC screening strategies fall in 2 broad categories: stool tests that primarily detect cancer, which include detection of occult blood or exfoliated DNA, and structural tests, such as flexible sigmoidoscopy, colonoscopy, and computed tomographic colonography, which are effective in detecting both cancer and premalignant lesions.[27]

Note: *CRC* stands for *colorectal cancer.*

6. According to the AUA, the presence of three or more red blood cells on a single, properly collected, noncontaminated urinalysis without evidence of infection is considered clinically significant microscopic hematuria.[28]

Note: *AUA* stands for *American Urological Association.*

Conclusion

Use normal sentence length to make your writing more readable. There is no scientific reason to write a long sentence. On the contrary, the science of reading ease indicates you should keep your sentence length moderate. We suggest the right length for medical writing is about 15 words average, with a maximum of about 25 words. Keep the subject and verb together in the first seven or eight words. Put the main point first.

In the next chapter, we consider word length and its effect on reading ease.

Notes

1. Orwell G, "Politics and the English Language," *Horizon* (April 1946). Available online, http://www.orwell.ru/library/essays/politics/english/e_polit/.
2. Watson, "Molecular Structure of Nucleic," *Nature* (see Intro, n. 11).
3. See for example Wydick, *Plain English for Lawyers*, 36 (see Intro, n. 8).
4. See for example Kimble, *Lifting the Fog of*, 71 (see Preface, n. 5); Wydick, *Plain English for Lawyers*, 36 (see Intro, n. 8).
5. See for example Brooks L, *Building Great Sentences: Exploring the Writer's Craft*, (Chantilly, VA: The Great Courses, 2008).
6. Cutts M, *Oxford Guide to Plain English*, 3rd ed. (Oxford: Oxford University Press, 2009), 2.
7. Alfandre D, Henning-Schumann J, "What is Wrong with Discharges Against Medical Advice (and How to Fix Them)," *JAMA* 310, no. 22 (2013): 2393.
8. Mannino D, Bust A, "Global Burden of COPD: Risk Factors, Prevalence, and Future Trends," *Lancet* 370 (September 2007): 765.

9. Rieder M, et al. "Effect of VKORC1 Haplotypes on Transcriptional Regulation and Warfarin Dose," *N Engl J Med* 352, no. 22 (2005): 2290.

10. Jorgensen T, et al. "Effect of Screening and Lifestyle Counselling on Incidence of Ischaemic Heart Disease in General Population: Inter99 Randomized Trial," *BMJ* 348 (2014), under "Introduction," http://www.bmj.com/content/348/bmj.g3617.

11. Bamman M, et al. "Exercise Biology and Medicine: Innovative Research to Improve Global Health," *Mayo Clinic Proc* 89, no. 2 (February 2014): 148.

12. Horne J, Flannery R, Usman S, "Adolescent Idiopathic Scoliosis: Diagnosis and Management," *Am Fam Phys* 89, no. 3 (February 2014): 194.

13. Greene, *Writing Science in Plain*, 18–21 (see Preface, n. 7).

14. Goldbart R, "Scientific Writing as an Art and as a Science," *Environmental Health* (March 2001): 22.

15. Alfandre, "What is Wrong with," 2393 (see chap. 1, n. 7).

16. Murray C, et. al. "Disability-adjusted Life Years (DALYs) for 291 Diseases and Injuries in 21 Regions, 1990–2010: A Systematic Analysis for the Global Burden of Disease Study 2010," *Lancet* 380 (December 2012): 2198.

17. Weinshilbourn R, "Inheritance and Drug Response," *N Engl J Med* 348, no. 6 (February 2003): 259.

18. Mallett S, et al. "Systematic Reviews of Diagnostic Tests in Cancer: Review of Methods and Reporting," *BMJ* 333 (August 2006), under "Reporting of Primary Study Details," http://www.bmj.com/content/333/7565/413.

19. Aakre B, et al. "Postoperative Acute Respiratory Distress Syndrome in Patients with Previous Exposure to Bleomycin," *Mayo Clinic Proc* 89, no. 2 (2014): 184–186.

20. Warner C, et al. "Identifying and Managing Posttraumatic Stress Disorder," *Am Fam Phys* 88, no. 12 (2013): 831.

21. Pelkowski T, Viera A, "Celiac Disease: Diagnosis and Management," *Am Fam Phys* 89, no. 2 (2014): 99.

22. Vinden C, et al. "Complications of Daytime Elective Laparoscopic Cholecystectomies Performed by Surgeons Who Operated the Night Before," *JAMA* 310, no. 17 (2013): 1840.

23. We found the term "($_{45}q_{15}$)," which refers to *the probability of death between 15 years and 60 years of age,* confusing.

24. Wang H, et al. "Age-specific and Sex-specific Mortality in 187 Countries, 1970–2010: A Systematic Analysis for the Global Burden of Disease Study 2010," *Lancet* 380 (2012): 2072.

25. Zineh I, Pacanowski M, Woodcock J, "Pharmacogenetics and Coumarin Dosing—Recalibrating Expectations," *N Engl J Med* 369, no. 24 (2013): 2274.

26. Jorgensen, "Effect of Screening and," under "Strengths and Limitations of Study," (see chap. 1, n. 10).

27. Bujanda L, et al. "Effect of Aspirin and Antiplatelet Drugs on the Outcome of the Fecal Immunochemical Test," *Mayo Clinic Proc* 88, no. 7 (2013): 683.

28. Sharp V, Barnes K, Erickson B, "Assessment of Asymptomatic Microscopic Hematuria in Adults," *Am Fam Phys* 88, no. 11 (2013): 748.

CHAPTER 2

Prefer the short word

If you want to influence your reader with your ideas, resist the temptation to use long Latin- or French-based words where shorter ones will do. Your message will be clearer and have much more impact.—Anne Greene, *Writing Science in Plain English*[1]

This chapter talks about how word length affects reading ease. If you want to write about medicine clearly and concisely, prefer the short word. Never use a big word just because you can. Use a big word when it helps you explain the science clearly and concisely. Impress people with your good ideas, not your big words.

A. Keep essential scientific terms; minimize other long words

What makes medical writing different from everyday speech? One difference is, everyday speech uses mostly one- or two-syllable words. Medical writing uses many words with three syllables or more.

We call long words that help you write science clearly and concisely, *essential scientific terms*. Minimize other long words. (We call a word, *a long word* if it has three syllables or more. But this doesn't include a two-syllable word that becomes a three-syllable word by adding a common ending, such as *-ed, -es,* or *–ing*. For example: *expand—expanded; transfuse—transfuses; report—reporting*.)

Essential scientific terms include names of diseases, medicines, chemicals and processes. They also include titles for studies and programs and other important scientific terms. How do you decide if a scientific term is *essential*? Every author needs to use their best judgment about this, but we think an essential scientific term meets four tests:

1. No shorter word serves just as well,
2. You can't paraphrase in a few short words,

3. Doctors and other medical scientists use the term consistently (i.e., exclusively), and
4. It's easy to look up in a standard reference.

Using these tests, *atrial fibrillation* qualifies as an essential scientific term since:

1. We can't think of a shorter word that serves just as well,
2. We can't paraphrase it in a few short words,
3. Doctors use it consistently, and
4. If you look up *atrial fibrillation* in a standard reference, you will find the right meaning right away.

Using these same tests, *pulmonary* does not qualify as an essential scientific term, since the word *lung* often serves just as well, and doctors use both terms.

Exercise 2.A. Keep essential scientific terms; minimize other long words
For each sentence:

1. Read it out loud and underline each <u>long word</u> (i.e., three syllables or more, not counting common word endings).
2. Double underline each word you consider an <u>essential scientific term</u>.
3. For any word you underlined only once, try to substitute a shorter word or paraphrase using a few shorter words. Make any other changes you can think of to improve reading ease.

Compare your answers to the Exercise Key in Appendix 3.

> **1. Therefore, it is not possible to determine whether all drug-eluting stents could benefit from short-term regimens of dual antiplatelet therapy based on the previous trials reported.[2]**
>
> **2. A careful assessment of the demographic evidence on the levels of age-specific mortality is an integral component of any Global Burden of Disease Study: such analyses require the sum of deaths from specific causes to equal the independently assessed level of mortality from all causes, for every age and sex group.[3]**
>
> **3. Most of the pharmacogenetic traits that were first identified were monogenic—that is, they involved only a single gene—and most were due to genetic polymorphisms; in other words, the allele or alleles responsible for the variation were relatively common.[4]**
>
> **4. Diagnostic accuracy is essential for good therapeutic treatment.[5]**

5. The 2 objectives of the study were (1) to examine the association between physical activity and dietary behavior and (2) to examine the potential combined effect of physical activity and dietary behavior on biological (eg, total cholesterol) and health (eg, waist circumference) markers.[6]

6. Assuming vasal disruption and occlusion have been adequately achieved during surgery, and assuming the patient adheres to using another contraceptive method while awaiting confirmation of sterility, true causes of vasectomy failure include recanalization (early and late) and, more rarely, aberrant anatomy (e.g., the presence of a third vas).[7]

B. Cite a common medical term once to avoid confusion

Many common medical terms don't qualify as an essential scientific term since they have a plain English equivalent or can be paraphrased in a few shorter words. Think of *urticara* (hives), *angioedema* (giant hives), *cardiovascular disease* (heart disease), *cerebrovascular disease* (blockage of arteries to the brain), and *ventricular hypertrophy* (heart wall thickening).

There may be times when you hesitate to write in plain English, because you feel it might confuse a reader if you *don't* use a common medical term. For example, consider the sentence: "The patient had <u>tachycardia</u> and <u>hypertension</u>, which are signs of <u>sympathochromaffin</u> system discharge <u>characteristic</u> of pain." None of the words underlined qualifies as an essential scientific term, but you might think a reader could be confused if you didn't use the terms *tachycardia, hypertension* and *sympathochromaffin system discharge*.

Where this is the case, we suggest writing in plain English, but stating the common medical term once in parentheses. For example: "The patient had a rapid heart rate (*tachycardia*) and high blood pressure (*hypertension*), which are signs of the 'fight-or-flight response' (*sympathochromaffin system discharge*) common for patients in pain." After you refer to the common medical term once, you are free to continue writing in plain English. This approach saves time for all readers, and helps reach the widest reasonable audience, but without unduly perpetuating *medicus incomprehensibilis*.

C. Write a compound word to promote reading ease and show how you pronounce it

One type of long word that often adds to *medicus incomprehensibilis* is the compound word. A *compound* is a word formed by combining two or more words, or a word plus a prefix. Medical writing uses many compounds formed from Latin or Greek root words. Try to handle compounds carefully, since:

- The longer the word, the lower the reading ease, and the less familiar it is likely to be.
- Any gap between how a word is written and how it is pronounced may slow down a reader.
- A reader may fail to see a word is a compound and puzzle over its meaning.
- An uncommon compound may be difficult to look up.

An occasional long compound may help explain the science clearly. But if you try to use every big word you know, it will lead to a severe case of *medicus incomprehensibilis*. You will lose many readers and waste other readers' time.

THREE MAIN TYPES OF COMPOUNDS

There are three main types of compounds: the *open compound*, the *closed compound*, and the *hyphenated compound*. With the *open compound*, words work together but are written as separate words. Examples include: *student nurse, 50 percent*, and *reference book*. Since the words aren't connected, you might not even think of them as compounds.

With the *closed compound*, words, or a word plus a prefix, are written as one word. Examples include: *multicell, hyperadrenergic, vasomotor* and *sinoatrial*. For some closed compounds, the meaning and syllable stress change. (For example, compare the compound, *straightforward* with the separate words, *straight* and *forward*. The compound has a different syllable stress and carries a slightly different meaning.) There is a general trend towards combining words to make new closed compounds (e.g., *on-line* becomes *online*).[8] In medical writing, this same trend can sometimes lead to ungainly long words that add to *medicus incomprehensibilis*.

With a *hyphenated compound*, words, or a word plus a prefix, are written together but separated by a hyphen. Examples are: *pre-menstrual, cost-effective, self-reported*. With the hyphenated compound, the component words are pronounced as separate words.

STANDARD USAGE FOR COMPOUNDS

For best reading ease, medical writing should follow standard usage regarding compounds and hyphenation. These rules are detailed and complex. For example, *The Chicago Manual of Style* contains 10 pages on compound words and hyphenation. Focusing on a few key guidelines can help a medical writer reduce *medicus incomprehensibilis*:

- Use caution in writing a word as a closed compound, unless that form is widely accepted and pronunciation and reading ease are not at stake.
- A well-placed hyphen can often make for easier reading.
- Words that can be misread should be hyphenated.
- Where no ambiguity would result, a hyphen is not mandatory. It may be better to write the word as an open compound.[9]

STRATEGIES FOR MANAGING COMPOUNDS

1. Consider paraphrasing
Often, you can paraphrase using shorter words.

2. Consider writing the word as an open compound
When you need to use a compound word, sometimes an open compound conveys the meaning just as well as a closed compound. It may also better reflect how you pronounce and improve clarity and reading ease. For example, the word, *ultra-rapid* is commonly written as a closed compound. But this tends to obscure how it is pronounced. It is four syllables long, which tends to lower reading ease.

We would prefer to write the word as an open compound, *ultra rapid*. To us, *ultra rapid* sounds like two words. We also don't see any special need to emphasize the connection between the parts. This way, it is easier to read and pronounce. The reading ease score also improves.

3. Consider writing the word as a hyphenated compound
Sometimes you can make a closed compound clearer by writing it as a hyphenated compound. Consider, the closed compound, *hyperadrenergic*. Since it is six syllables long, it will lower the reading ease in any sentence where it appears. This compound joins the words, *hyper-* and *adrenergic*, but you can't find *hyperadrenergic* in Stedman's Medical Dictionary. Instead you have to look up the two parts. *Adrenergic* is itself a closed compound made up of Latin and Greek roots.[10] We can make things clearer by writing this word as a hyphenated compound, *hyper-adrenergic*. (Because people think of *hyper-* as a prefix, we would not try to write *hyper adrenergic* as an open compound.)

Or, consider another closed compound, *psychomotor*. Anyone not familiar with this word might try to say, *psy-CHOM-o-tor,* as though it rhymed with *barometer*. As a result, they also might miss that it is formed from the words *psycho* and *motor*. The right way to pronounce this word is, *PSYcho-MOtor.* It sounds like two words, with the stress at the beginning of each word. We think it would be clearer to write it as *psycho-motor*. This helps close the gap between how we write and how we speak. It should be easier to read and understand.

Table 2-1 shows examples of some other closed compounds we would prefer to write as hyphenated compounds to help show meaning and pronunciation more clearly.

Table 2-1. **Hyphenate to show how you pronounce**

Closed compound	Hyphenated compound
postherpetic neuralgia	post-herpetic neuralgia
multinational	multi-national
antiviral	anti-viral
nonfatal	non-fatal

Each of these examples might confuse a reader on first reading, if only for an instant. For example, somebody might easily misread the word *postherpetic* as *POS-therpetic*. Writing this word as a hyphenated compound, *post-herpetic* helps the reader better see the units of meaning.

Some of the same considerations apply to prefixes. Consider the words *decontaminate* or *deactivate*. We pronounce them as if they were written as *D-contaminate* and *D-activate*. (We don't say *DECK-kon-ta-mi-nate* or *DEAK-ti-vate*.) For an international medical audience, we think it would be better to write *de-contaminate* and *de-activate*.

WHEN WOULDN'T WE HYPHENATE?

It takes judgment to decide when to use a hyphen. We wouldn't create a hyphenated compound when an open compound conveys the meaning just as clearly. We would hesitate to hyphenate an essential scientific term. We also wouldn't hyphenate when a closed compound meets three tests:

1. It is fairly short—usually three syllables or less,
2. Writing it as a closed compound is well-accepted in *common* usage, and
3. There is little chance a reader might mispronounce the word.

Guided by these principles, we would not hyphenate *prefix, react, prototype, ultrasound* or *phenotype*. There may be other cases where you choose not to hyphenate a compound word. But you should always try to write a compound word as clearly as you can to help reduce *medicus incomprehensibilis*.

Some journals may have a house style for writing compounds that differs from the advice we give here. If you take care to write compounds clearly, but an editor or reviewer insists on using their house style, by all means, defer to their judgment.

Exercise 2.C. Write a compound word to promote reading ease and show how you pronounce it
While you're in Stockholm to accept your Nobel Prize, you dine with other prize winners who speak English, but not as well as you. One of them asks for your help to pronounce the words underlined in the examples.

1. For each word underlined, either add a hyphen to help show the word's meaning or pronunciation, or tell why you think adding a hyphen wouldn't be helpful.
2. Revise to make any other changes you can think of to improve reading ease.

Compare your answers to the Exercise Key in Appendix 3.

1. <u>Predefining</u> a threshold value for heart rate is difficult because it must be individualized in the context of the patient's overall <u>hemodynamic</u> status and any <u>preexisting</u> <u>comorbidities</u>.[11]

2. For example, the results of the Burden of Lung Disease (BOLD) study—a <u>multinational</u> investigation of the <u>prevalence</u> of COPD using a standard methodology and reported in this issue of *The Lancet*, show that one of the highest <u>prevalences</u> of COPD was recorded in South Africa, a country that also has a high <u>prevalence</u> of tuberculosis.[12]

3. Although a recent study showed that <u>genotype</u>-guided dosing led to superior control of <u>anticoagulation</u>, the finding was based on a comparison with a <u>nonrandomized</u>, real-world parallel control group.[13]

4. Flavonoids are naturally occurring <u>bioactive</u> compounds that represent a constituent of fruits and vegetables, beyond calorie and <u>macronutrient</u> content, that could potentially influence body weight.[14]

5. One of the identified causes of delay in ET is <u>multimodal</u> imaging.[15]

Note: *ET* stands for *endovascular therapy*.

6. The recommended modalities are <u>photodynamic</u> therapy, <u>radiofrequency</u> ablation, or <u>endoscopic</u> mucosal <u>resection</u>.[16]

D. Omit any unnecessary word ending

Languages sometimes change a word ending to show how the word functions in a sentence. For example, in modern English, we use *s* to show plural, and *'s* to show possession or connection. We also have Latin-origin words that show possession or connection using other endings: *gene/gen<u>etic</u>, molecule/molecul<u>ar</u>, practice/ practical, muscle/musc<u>ular</u>.*

Languages tend to lose endings over time. We may ask, is it clearer or more correct to say *math<u>ematical</u> calculation* or *math calculation*? In our view, both are clear and correct, but *math* is more concise. It sounds less formal, but not distracting or un-professional. Since using *math* helps improve reading ease, we would prefer it. Respecting a colleague's time, by writing as clearly and concisely as possible, is always the most professional way to write.

Which endings do you need to convey your meaning clearly and concisely? Your judgment may be as good as ours or better. Whenever you can reasonably leave off a word ending, it helps improve reading ease.

Exercise 2.D. Omit any unnecessary word ending
For each sentence, we underlined a word ending that shows possession or connection *(e.g., cell/cellular; gene/genetic)*.

1. Read the sentence out loud. Do you think it would work to delete the ending and just use the root word? Or else, to use a simpler word? Why or why not?
2. Revise the sentence, making any other changes you can think of to improve reading ease.

Compare your answers to the Exercise Key in Appendix 3.

> **1. Given that this was an observational study, unmeasured confounding or hidden bias might exist.**[17]
>
> **2. However, poverty is regarded as a surrogate measure for many factors that subsequently increase the risk of COPD, such as poor nutritional status, crowding, exposure to pollutants including high work exposures and high smoking rates (in countries of low and middle income), poor access to health care, and early respiratory infections.**[18]
>
> **3. The concept of pharmacogenetics originated from the clinical observation that there were patients with very high or very low plasma or urinary drug concentrations, followed by the realization that the biochemical traits leading to this variation were inherited.**[19]
>
> **4. Benefit from combined mammography and breast physical examination screening was found in women aged 50–64, but not in women aged 40–49.**[20]
>
> **5. If familial cardiomyopathy is suggested on the basis of history, genetic testing and referral to a genetic counselor should be considered.**[21]
>
> **6. Dosing must be tailored to the patient's symptoms and inflammatory markers because up to 13% of patients required higher initial doses.**[22]

E. Avoid the noun string

One writing habit that often involves long words and low reading ease is the *noun string*. A noun string is a group of nouns and their modifiers put into long strings.[23] Sometimes, one noun modifies another noun. Here are a few examples: *early childhood thought disorder misdiagnosis, pre-adolescent hyperactivity diagnosis,* and *medication maintenance level evaluation procedures.*[24] When a sentence uses more than three nouns in a row, it becomes harder to read.[25] The reader can't see at first glance which word in the string is important.

WHEN SHOULD YOU USE A NOUN STRING?

You may want to use a short, familiar noun string to help name a complex concept in just a few words. Otherwise, avoid long strings that are not already well known.[26] Avoid creating a new noun string.[27]

Exercise 2.E. Avoid the noun string
For each sentence:

1. Read it out loud and underline each <u>noun string</u>.
2. Revise the sentence to eliminate the noun string. Make any other changes you can think of to improve reading ease.

Compare your answers to the Exercise Key in Appendix 3.

> **1. The study by Vinden et al provides direct evidence from patient outcomes that operating the night before is not associated with increased complications for elective laparoscopic cholecystectomies performed the following day.**[28]
>
> **2. Performance is assessed in terms of rigorous out-of-sample predictive validity testing based on the root-mean-squared error of the log of the age-specific death rates, the percentage of time that trend is accurately predicted, and the coverage of the uncertainty intervals (UIs).**[29]
>
> **3. By targeting VKOR, the post-translational modification of the vitamin K-dependent blood-coagulation proteins is impaired.**[30]

Note: *VKOR* stands for *vitamin K epoxide reductase.*

> **4. All participants with an unhealthy lifestyle had individually tailored lifestyle counselling at all visits (at baseline and after one and three years); those at high risk of ischaemic heart disease, according to pre-defined criteria, were furthermore offered six sessions of group based lifestyle counselling on smoking cessation, diet, and physical activity.**[31]
>
> **5. As in the original CMS readmission model derivation, patients who were discharged and then died before being rehospitalized were not counted as "failures"; that is, they were included in the analysis but not assigned a readmission event.**[32]

6. Tick paralysis, which results from gravid female bites, is a toxin-mediated ascending paralysis that generally resolves after tick removal.[33]

F. Don't be afraid to start a sentence with *and* or *but*

Medical articles often start a sentence by using a long conjunction, such as *furthermore, nevertheless,* or *however,* in order to continue an idea started in the previous sentence. It would improve reading ease to substitute *and, but,* or some other short conjunction, but you almost never see this. This complete aversion to starting a sentence with *and* or *but* is unwarranted.[34] Sometimes *and* or *but* sounds fine; sometimes it doesn't.

Exercise 2.F. Don't be afraid to start a sentence with and *or* but
For each exerpt:

1. Read it out loud and underline the long conjunction that starts the last sentence.
2. Try replacing that long conjunction with *and, but,* or some other short word, and read it out loud again. How does it sound to you?
3. Revise to make any other changes you can think of to improve reading ease.

Compare your answers to the Exercise Key in Appendix 3.

1. Because patients with sepsis have a wide range of sympathetic activation and responsiveness, giving a fixed dose of a β-blocker would probably be less effective and potentially harmful if given to all patients. Furthermore, because adrenergic stress persists as long as the external stress (eg, infection or injury), treatment was continued for the entire intensive care unit stay.[35]

2. The period since 1970 has been characterized by substantial heterogeneity in mortality transitions. Life expectancy in Japanese women in 2010 was 85.9 years, and is probably higher in 2012. However, the gain in the past 40 years was only 11 years, compared with total improvements of two to three times more in other parts of Asia (eg, the Maldives), the Middle East (especially Oman), and Latin American (eg, Bolivia, Peru, and Guatemala).[36]

3. Our analysis does not address the issue of whether a precise initial dose of warfarin translates into improved clinical end points, such as a reduction in the time needed to achieve a stable therapeutic INR, fewer INRs that are out of range, and a reduced incidence of

bleeding or thromboembolic events. However, our study lays important groundwork for a prospective trial and suggests that such a trial should be powered to detect the benefits of incorporating pharmacogenetic information into the dose algorithm for patients who require high or low doses—the subgroups in our study for whom dose estimates based on the pharmacogenetic algorithm differed significantly from those based on the clinical algorithm.[37]

4. Studies are observational in nature, prone to various biases, and report two linked measures summarizing the performance in participants with disease (sensitivity) and without (specificity). In addition, there is more variation between studies in the methods, manufacturers, procedures, and outcome measurement scales used to assess test accuracy than in randomized controlled trials, which generally causes marked heterogeneity in results.[38]

5. This addresses not only the challenge of selection but also several other challenges (eg, availability and recognition). However, participants noted several liabilities with this approach, including lack of subspecialty specificity, additional uncompensated effort or institutional expense, and potential for overreliance on the system.[39]

6. This study found that older patients who had severe neurocardiogenic syncope (average of seven syncopal episodes in the previous two years and asystolic pauses averaging 11 seconds) had a decreased time to first syncopal event after a pacemaker was implanted. However, this study was a manufacturer-funded trial and did not report the total syncopal burden or number of falls.[40]

G. Avoid using a high percentage of long words

Common English tends to use an occasional long word. Medical writing needs to use essential scientific terms to help the reader understand the science. This probably means using more long words than common English. In both cases, common English and medical writing, the occasional well-chosen long word is probably not a problem. The reader might not even notice.[41]

By contrast, some medical articles use far too many non-essential long words. A high percentage of long words is a symptom of severe *medicus incomprehensibilis*. Good science, expressed using essential scientific terms, helps to inform and persuade the reader. It may even impress them. Inflated diction that serves no scientific purpose usually fails to impress.[42]

Exercise 2.G. Avoid using a high percentage of long words
1. Underline each <u>long word</u> in the excerpt. Double underline each <u>*essential scientific term*</u>.

2. Compute long words as a percentage of total words. (# long words/270 words = ___ %)
3. Revise to minimize long words but keep essential scientific terms. Break up any long sentence and make other changes to improve reading ease.
4. Compute a new percentage of long words for the revised excerpt. How big a change did you achieve? Do you feel your revision improved reading ease?

Compare your answers to the Exercise Key in Appendix 3.

> In a majority of cases, metabolism that is mediated by cytochrome P-450 represents a deactivation pathway. For some drugs, however, oxidation leads to conversion of a prodrug into an active compound. A prime example is codeine (metabolized by CYP2D6); other examples include clopidogrel (metabolized by CYP3A4), cyclophosphamide (metabolized by CYP2B6) and tamoxifen (metabolized by CYP2D6). The major pathway of codeine consists of glucuronidation and N-demethylation, whereas the CYP2D6-mediated O-demethylation to produce morphine is a minor reaction. Nevertheless, the latter is a crucial step in bioactivation, since the affinity of codeine for the μ-opioid receptor is only 1/200 to 1/3000 that of morphine. Previous studies have shown that the effects of codeine—analgesic, respiratory, psychomotor, and miotic—are markedly attenuated in people with poor metabolism of CYP2D6. On the other hand, people with ultrarapid metabolism, such as the patient described by Gasche et al. in this issue of the *Journal*, produce greater amounts of morphine from codeine and therefore may experience exaggerated pharmacologic effects in response to regular doses of codeine. Similar effects, albeit less dramatic, have been described in patients with ultrarapid metabolism of CYP2D6 in response to routine doses of hydrocodone or oxycodone, which are other opioids requiring CYP2D6 mediated activation. These reports clearly illustrate the effect of CYP2D6 genetic polymorphisms on the action of codeine, ranging from virtually no effect in patients with poor metabolism to severe toxic effects in those with ultrarapid metabolism. To put these observations into perspective, these extremes of response might be relevant for some 10 to 20 percent of whites who have phenotypes associated with either poor metabolism or ultrarapid metabolism.[43]

Conclusion

The two easiest things you can do to make your writing more readable are to use normal sentence length and prefer the short word. Just as there is no scientific reason to write a long sentence, there is no scientific reason to use many non-essential long words. On the contrary, the science of reading ease indicates you should prefer the shortest word that does the job. When you can master these two lessons, you will have gone a long way toward improving reading ease.

Notes

1. Greene, *Writing Science in Plain*, 30 (see Preface, n. 7).
2. Feres F, et al. "Three vs. Twelve Months of Dual Antiplatelet Therapy after Zotarolimus-eluting Stents: The OPTIMIZE Randomized Trial," *JAMA* 310, no. 23 (2013): 1517.
3. Wang, "Age-specific and Sex-specific Mortality," 2071–2072 (see chap. 1, n. 24).
4. Weinshilbourn, "Inheritance and Drug Response," 529 (see chap. 1, n. 17).
5. Mallett, "Systematic Reviews of Diagnostic," under "Introduction," (see chap. 1, n. 18).
6. Loprinzi P, Smit E, Mahoney S, "Physical Activity and Dietary Behavior in US Adults and Their Combined Influence on Health," *Mayo Clinic Proc* 89, no. 2 (February 2014): 190.
7. Rayala B, Viera A, "Common Questions about Vasectomy," *Am Fam Phys* 88, no. 11(2013): 759.
8. *Chicago Manual of Style*, 15th ed., s.v. § 7.84.
9. Ibid. §§ 7.84–7.90.
10. Adren [L. *ad*, to + *ren*, kidney] + [G. *Ergon*, work]; *Stedman's Medical Dictionary*, ed. 28, s.vv. "Hyper," "Adrenergic."
11. Morelli, "Effect of Heart Rate," 1689 (see chap. 1, Table 1-1).
12. Mannino, "Global Burden of COPD," 767 (see chap. 1, n. 8).
13. Pirmohamed M, et al. "A Randomized Trial of Genotype-Guided Dosing of Warfarin," *N Engl J Med* 369, no. 24 (2013): 2295.
14. Bertoia M, et al. "Dietary Flavonoid Intake and Weight Maintenance: Three Prospective Cohorts of 124,086 US Men and Women Followed for up to 24 Years," *BMJ* 352, no. i17 (2016), under "Introduction," http://dx.doi.org/10.1136/bmj.i17.
15. Singh B, et al. "Endovascular Therapy for Acute Ischemic Stroke: A Systematic Review and Meta-Analysis," *Mayo Clinic Proc* 88, no. 10 (2013): 1064.
16. Zimmerman T, "Common Questions about Barrett's Esophagus," *Am Fam Phys* 89, no. 2 (2014): 96.
17. Vigen R, et al. "Association of Testosterone Therapy with Mortality, Myocardial Infarction, and Stroke in Men with Low Testosterone Levels," *JAMA* 310, no. 17 (2013): 1834.
18. Mannino, "Global Burden of COPD," 769 (see chap. 1, n. 8).
19. Weinshilbourn, "Inheritance and Drug Response," 529 (see chap. 1, n. 17).
20. Miller A, et al. "Twenty-Five Year Follow-up for Cancer Incidence and Mortality of the Canadian National Breast Screening Study: Randomized Screening Trials," *BMJ* 348 (2014) under "Introduction," http://www.bmj.com/content/348/bmg.g366.
21. Dunlay S, Pereira N, Kushawaha S, "Contemporary Strategies in the Diagnosis and Management of Heart Failure," *Mayo Clinic Proc* 89, no. 5 (May 2014): 663.
22. Caylor T, Perkins A, "Recognition and Management of Polymyalgia Rheumatica and Giant Cell Arteritis," *Am Fam Phys* 88, no. 10 (November 2013): 678.
23. Greene, *Writing Science in Plain*, 35–36 (see Preface, n. 7).
24. Williams, *Style: Lessons in Clarity*, 70 (see Preface, n. 8).
25. See for example Follett W, *Modern American Usage*, (1966), quoted in *A Dictionary of Modern Legal Usage*, Garner B, (New York: Oxford University Press, 1987), s.v. "Noun Plague," 380.
26. Greene, *Writing Science in Plain*, 35–36 (see Preface, n. 7).
27. Williams, *Style: Lessons in Clarity*, 69–70 (see Preface, n. 8).
28. Zinner M, Fresichlag J, "Surgeons, Sleep and Patient Safety," *JAMA* 310, no. 17 (2013): 1808.

29. Murray, "Disability-Adjusted Life Years," 2200 (see chap. 1, n. 16).

30. Furie B, "Do Pharmacogenetics Have a Role in the Dosing of Vitamin K Antagonists?" *N Eng J Med* 367, no. 24 (2013): 2345.

31. Jorgensen, "Effect of Screening and," under "Intervention," (see chap. 1, n. 10).

32. Hummel S, et al. "Impact of Prior Admissions on 30-day Readmission in Medicare Heart Failure Inpatients," *Mayo Clinic Proc* 89, no. 5 (May 2014): 624.

33. Juckett G, "Arthropod Bites," *Am Fam Phys* 88, no. 12 (2013): 844.

34. *A Dictionary of Modern,* Garner, s.vv. "And," "But" (see chap. 2, n. 25).

35. Pinsky M, "Is there a Role for β-blockage in Septic Shock?" *JAMA* 310, no. 16 (2013): 1677.

36. Wang, "Age-specific and Sex-specific Mortality," under "Discussion" (see chap. 1, n. 24).

37. The International Warfarin Pharmacogenetics Consortium, "Estimation of the Warfarin Dose with Clinical and Pharmacogenetic Data," *N Eng J Med* 360, no. 8 (2009): 760.

38. Mallett, "Systematic Reviews of Diagnostic," under "Introduction" (see chap. 1, n. 18).

39. Cook D, Sorensen K, Wilkinson J, "Value and Process of Curbside Consultations in Clinical Practice: A Grounded Theory Study," *Mayo Clinic Proc* 89, no. 5 (2014): 610.

40. Denay K, Johanson M, "Common Questions About Pacemakers," *Am Fam Phys* 89, no. 4 (2014): 281.

41. Kimble, *Lifting the Fog of Legalese*, 164 (see Preface, n. 5).

42. Ibid., 72.

43. Caraco Y, "Genes and the Response to Drugs," *N Eng J Med* 351, no. 27 (2004): 2868.

CHAPTER 3

Omit any needless word

The ability to simplify means to eliminate the unnecessary so that the necessary may speak.—Hans Hoffman[1]

Plain English writing means avoiding or omitting needless words that contribute to *medicus incomprehensibilis*. In this chapter, we give exercises for you to practice spotting and eliminating needless words. We also point out a few common markers for needless words: *of* and *that*.

A. Spot and omit needless words

The next exercise asks you to practice spotting and omitting needless words.

Exercise 3.A. Spot and omit needless words
For each excerpt:

1. Read it out loud. Strike any word you think unnecessary and do minor rearranging or editing, as needed.
2. Count the number of words you struck and calculate the percent reduction. (For example, if you strike 3 words from a 30-word sentence, the reduction is 3/30 = 10.0%.)
3. Revise to make any other changes you can think of to improve reading ease.

Compare your answers to the Exercise Key in Appendix 3.

> **1. In our study, we hypothesized that a heart rate range between 80/min to 94/min was a sufficient compromise between improving cardiac performance and preserving systemic hemodynamics.[2]**

> **2. Although the definition states that this effect is in response to noxious particles or gases, such as those in tobacco smoke, there is also some evidence that infections can have an important role in the presence of chronic inflammation in the lung.[3]**

3. In the multiple linear regression analysis adjusted for clinically important covariates, four of the five common haplotypes were found to be independently associated with the warfarin dose ($P \leq 0.05$) (Table 1).[4]

4. With the emergence of new direct acting antivirals, the treatment paradigm for hepatitis C virus (HCV) infection is currently undergoing its greatest change since the discovery of the virus 25 years ago.[5]

5. Both dietary and physical activity behavior are independent predictors of numerous health outcomes among adults.[6]

6. For historical reasons, the American Indian/Alaska Native population is particularly at risk of health and health care disparities. We examined national data to understand how American Indians/Alaska Natives use the health care system. To visualize the comparison we employed an "ecology of health care" model which uses a relative box size to indicate differences between populations. We compared American Indians/Alaska Natives with the remaining U.S. population on self-rated poor health (see accompanying figure).

This analysis reveals, as expected, the American Indian/Alaska Native population to be significantly more rural and impoverished than the rest of the U.S. population. In addition, American Indians/Alaska Natives rate their health as poorer, yet they access the health care system less often than the rest of the U.S. population. When they do access the health care system, they more often enter through emergency departments. Despite poorer health of American Indians/Alaska Natives, the rates of primary care visits and hospitalizations are similar to the rest of the U.S. population.[7]

B. Omit the needless *of*

The word *of* is a marker for wordiness. If you search for the word *of* in your draft, you can often find a way to omit a few needless words (either *of* or other words). Test this tip for yourself in the following exercise.

Exercise 3.B. Omit the needless of
For each sentence:

1. Read it out loud and underline the word *of* wherever it appears.
2. Revise to eliminate *of* or other needless words you see. Make any other changes you can think of to improve reading ease.

Compare your answers to the Exercise Key in Appendix 3.

1. The objective of our study was to conduct a randomized, multi-center clinical trial to assess the effect of CPAP treatment on blood

pressure values and nocturnal blood pressure patterns of patients with resistant hypertension and OSA.[8]

Note: *CPAP* stands for *continuous positive airway pressure. OSA* stands for *obstructive sleep apnea.*

2. Estimates of the number of deaths in children younger than 5 years from the UNPD are substantially higher than are our estimations; for 2005–2010, their estimates are 8 million deaths higher (1–6 million per year).[9]

Note: *UNPD* stands for *United Nations Population Division.*

3. Recurring themes in pharmacogenetics include the presence of a few relatively common variant alleles of genes encoding proteins important in drug response, a larger number of much less frequent variant alleles, and striking differences in the types and frequencies of alleles among different populations and ethnic groups. [10]

4. The quality of the studies varied considerably; many studies were old, and few of the published studies provided sufficient detail to replicate the intervention used.[11]

5. At the time that the 2004 algorithm was published, there were 2 available rigorous evidence-base reviews of the treatment of RLS/WED prepared under the auspices of the Standards of Practice Committee of the American Academy of Sleep Medicine.[12]

Note: *RLS/WED* stands for *restless legs syndrome/Willis-Ekbom disease.*

6. Systemic symptoms (low-grade fever, fatigue, malaise, and weight loss) occur in 30% to 50% of patients.[13]

C. Omit the needless *that*

Like *of*, the word *that* can also be a marker for wordiness. In some languages, you must use the equivalent of *that* to start a dependent clause (e.g., *daβ* in German, *que* in French or Spanish, что in Russian, or *ka* in Latvian). But in English, sometimes you need it and sometimes you don't. If you don't need it, it's best to leave it out.

Table 3-1 shows examples of short sentences that are clear without using *that* to introduce a clause. In other cases, you may need *that* to avoid confusion. But, where this is the case, consider whether the sentence might be too long and contain too many ideas. Perhaps, rather than keeping *that*, it would be better to split up the long sentence to make shorter sentences.

Table 3-1. **You don't always need** *that* **to start a clause**

With that	*Without* that
The intern suggested *that* Raul needed a CAT scan.	The intern suggested Raul needed a CAT scan.
The test confirmed *that* Natalia was pregnant.	The test confirmed Natalia was pregnant.

Exercise 3.C. Omit the needless that
For each excerpt:

1. Read it out loud and underline the word *that* each time it occurs. Then decide whether you think it's necessary.
2. Strike out any *that* or any other words you think unnecessary. (If you need to, do other minor editing or re-arranging to make this work.)
3. Then revise to make any other changes you can think of to improve reading ease.

Compare your answers to the Exercise Key in Appendix 3.

1. Prevalence studies estimate that 38,054 patients had a diagnosis of a primary malignant brain tumor in the United States in 2010.[14]

2. Deaths assigned to causes that are not likely to underlie causes of death have been reassigned with standardized algorithms.[15]

3. Other states have simplified or eliminated special prescribing rules (such as those requiring the use of triplicate prescription pads) that were designed to control and monitor prescribing but that had the (presumably unintended) effect of discouraging all prescribing of controlled substances.[16]

4. It has therefore been clear for some time that more effective and tolerable treatment regiments for HCV are needed.[17]

Note: *HCV* stands for *hepatitis C virus*.

5. A more recent analysis by Goyal et al revealed that both admission and post-admission hyperglycemia (admission glucose level ≤ 3.8 mmo/L) could predict 30-day death rate in patients with AMI.[18]

Note: *AMI* stands for *acute myocardial infarction*.

6. Overt hyperthyroidism that is inadequately treated is associated with an increased risk of adverse maternal and neonatal outcomes (Table 4).[19]

Conclusion

This chapter covered the tip, *Omit any needless word.* This seems obvious but we all need a reminder from time to time.

In the last three chapters, we looked at tips for improving your reading ease score. In the next part of the book, we shift our focus to the concept of vivid language.

Notes

1. Williams, *Style: Lessons in Clarity,* 111 (see Preface, n. 8).
2. Morelli, "Effect of Heart Rate," 1689 (see chap. 1, Table 1-1).
3. Mannino, "Global Burden of COPD," 766 (see chap. 1, n. 8).
4. Rieder, "Effect of VKORC1 Haplotypes," 2289 (see chap. 1, n. 9).
5. Feeney E, Chung R, "Antiviral Treatment of Hepatitis C," *BMJ* 349 (2014), under "Introduction," http://www.bmj.com/content/349/bmj.g3308.
6. Loprinzi, "Physical Activity and Dietary," 190 (see chap. 2, n. 6).
7. Elise A G, et al. "Ecology of Health Care: The Need to Address Low Utilization in American Indians/Alaska Natives," *Am Fam Phys* 79, no. 3 (2014): 217.
8. Martinez-Garcia M, et al. "Effect of CPAP on Blood Pressure in Patients with Obstructive Sleep Apnea and Resistant Hypertension: The HIPARCO Randomized Clinical Trial," *JAMA* 310, no. 22 (2013): 2408.
9. Wang, "Age-specific and Sex-specific Mortality," 2087 (see chap. 1, n. 24).
10. Weinshilbourn, "Inheritance and Drug Response," 532 (see chap. 1, n. 17).
11. Jorgensen, "Effect of Screening and," *BMJ,* under "Introduction" (see chap. 1, n. 10).
12. Silber M, et al. "Willis-Ekbom Disease Foundation Revised Consensus Statement on the Management of Restless Legs Syndrome," *Mayo Clinic Proc* 88, no. 9 (2013): 978.
13. Caylor, "Recognition and Management of," 677 (see chap. 2, n. 22).
14. Omuro A, DeAngelis L, "Glioblastoma and Other Malignant Gliomas: A Clinical Review," *JAMA* 310, no. 17 (2013): 1842.
15. Murray, "Disability-Adjusted Life Years," 2200 (see chap. 1, n. 16).
16. Quill T, Meier D, "The Big Chill: Inserting the DEA into End-of-Life Care," *N Eng J Med* 354, no. 1 (2006): 1–2.
17. Feeney, "Antiviral Treatment of Hepatitis," under "Indirect Acting Antivirals—Interferon Alfa and Ribavirin," (see chap. 3, n. 5).
18. Yang S, et al. "Association of Dysglycemia and All-Cause Mortality Across the Spectrum of Coronary Artery Disease," *Mayo Clinic Proc* 88, no. 9 (2013): 938.
19. Carney L, Quinlan J, West J, "Thyroid Disease in Pregnancy," *Am Fam Phys* 89, no. 4 (2014): 276.

2

USE VIVID LANGUAGE

Belief is nothing but a more vivid, lively, forcible, firm, steady conception of an object, than what the imagination alone is ever able to attain.—David Hume[1]

The second concept for writing clearly and concisely is, *Use vivid language*. Using *vivid language* means using language that is *clear, detailed, powerful, full of life,* or *strikingly alive*. Good writing is lively. We trace the word *vivid* to the Latin words for *alive, spirited* or *animated*.[2]

Medical writing is naturally interesting since it involves human life. The word *biology* means the "study of life."[3] A good medical science article should reflect the natural vitality of the subject. It should propel the reader along so they learn faster, better and easier. No medical writer should ever do anything to destroy this natural vitality by trying to make their writing dull and boring.

This is not to say a medical article should be *poetic, thrilling,* or *entertaining,* the way other types of writing sometimes are. After all, a doctor or other scientist reads a journal to learn, not to be entertained. Still, an author should never seek the opposite extreme by boring, confusing, or frustrating a reader with dull and barely readable prose. Yet, sadly, some authors seem to do just that.

Up until now, our tips on improving reading ease haven't considered scientific content. From now on, they will deal more and more with scientific content, but they may not always improve reading ease.

In the next three chapters, we give tips on making medical writing more vivid.

4. Prefer active voice
5. Prefer concrete language
6. Observe the 1066 principle

Notes

1. Hume D, "An Enquiry Concerning Human Understanding: Skeptical Solution of these Doubts," in *The Harvard Classics*, ed. Charles W. Eliot (New York: Collier) 37: 344.
2. The word *vivid* comes from Latin *vividus* (animated, spirited), from *vivere* (to live), akin to *vita* (life), Ancient Greek *βίος* (bíos, life); *Wiktionary, s.v.* "Vivid," (accessed January 4, 2015) https://en.wiktionary.org/wiki/vivid.
3. The term *biology* (Bio- + -logy) is a modern term coined by taking its components from Ancient Greek βίος (bíos, bio-, life) + -λογία (-logía, -logy, branch of study, to speak). This term or analogous terms arose in different European languages around 1800. The word βιολογία did not exist in Ancient Greek. *Wiktionary, s.v.* "Biology," (accessed January 4, 2015) https://en.wiktionary.org/wiki/vivid.

CHAPTER 4

Prefer active voice

Too often, aspiring professionals think they join the club only when they write in the club's most complex technical language. It is an exclusionary style that erodes the trust a civil society depends on, especially in a world where information and expertise are now the means to power and control. It is true some research can never be made clear to merely intelligent lay readers—but less often than many researchers think.
—Joseph Williams[1]

Traditional medical writing over-uses passive voice. If you want to write vividly, prefer writing in active voice. Use passive voice, sparingly, only when it helps you write clearly and concisely.

A sentence in active voice reflects the way we talk to other people every day, so a reader finds it easy to follow. It also sounds more direct and vigorous than one written in passive voice. Using active voice as a habit makes for forceful writing. This is true, not just with a writing concerned mainly with action, but for any kind of writing. When you revise a sentence in active voice, it usually becomes shorter.[2]

What do the terms *active voice* and *passive voice* mean?

In case you need it, here's a quick refresher on active and passive voice. The term *voice* describes whether the subject of the sentence is *doing* the action or *receiving* the action. When the subject *does* the action, the verb is in active voice. When the subject *receives* the action, the verb is in passive voice.[3] Table 4-1 shows examples of passive and active voice.

Some sentences are neither active nor passive, since the subject neither does, nor receives any action. Such a sentence may describe a state of being or a state of possession.

Table 4-1. **Examples of passive and active voice**

Passive	Active
Patients and clinicians were recruited from 7 clinical sites.[i]	We recruited patients and clinicians from 7 clinical sites.
The final analysis was performed according to the intention-to-treat principle after the enrollment period ended for the study.[ii]	We analyzed the data according to the intention-to-treat principle after the enrollment period ended for the study.
Studies of HIV in women were either routinely undertaken within populations of female sex workers or included a substantial number of them.[iii]	A study of HIV in women often covered a study group made up of only female sex workers, or included a large number of them.

[i]Kravitz R, et al. "Patient Engagement Programs for Recognition and Initial Treatment of Depression in Primary Care: A Randomized Trial," *JAMA* 310, no. 17 (2013): 1819.

[ii]Annane D, et al. "Effects of Fluid Resuscitation with Colloids vs. Crystalloids on Mortality in Critically Ill Patients Presenting with Hypovolemic Shock: The CRISTAL Randomized Trial," *JAMA* 310, no. 17 (2013): 1812.

[iii]Beyrer, "An Action Agenda for," *Lancet,* under "Introduction" (see chap. 4, n. 6).

A. Identify active and passive voice

How do you identify a sentence written in passive voice? A passive sentence has two basic features, although both may not appear in every passive sentence. The first is a form of the verb *to be* (for example: *is, are, was, were, has been, will have been, would be, etc*). The second is a past participle (generally, with an *-ed* ending).[4] (See Glossary.)

The three examples in Table 4-1 each use a form of the verb *to be* and a past participle: in the first example, *were recruited*. In the second, *was performed*. In the third, *were . . . undertaken*.

Exercise 4.A. Identify active and passive voice
For each sentence:

1. Read it out loud and underline the <u>subject once</u> and the <u>verb twice</u>. Draw braces around any {past participle}.
2. Is the sentence active, passive or neither?

Compare your answers to the Exercise Key in Appendix 3.

1. For those patients randomized to CPAP treatment, optimal CPAP pressure was titrated in the sleep laboratory on a second night by

an auto CPAP device (REMstar Pro M series with C-Flex, Philips Respironics) within a period of less than 15 days after the diagnostic study to obtain a fixed CPAP pressure value, according to a previous validation by the Spanish Sleep Network.[5]

Note: *CPAP* stands for *continuous positive airway pressure.*

2. A meta-analysis of data from 14 countries reported that transgender female sex workers had a higher burden of HIV (27%) than other transgender women (15%), male (15%), and female sex workers (5%).[6]

3. Warfarin binds to albumin, and only about 3% is free and pharmacologically active.[7]

4. After entry, the 9.6 kb viral genome undergoes cytoplasmic translation into a single polypeptide, which is subsequently cleaved into 10 viral proteins—three structural and seven non-structural.[8]

5. This sex difference is not clearly understood.[9]

6. Ticagrelor is recommended for combination therapy with aspirin in patients who have acute coronary syndrome (unstable angina, non-ST elevation myocardial infarction, or ST elevation myocardial infarction) to reduce death from cardiovascular causes.[10]

B. Revise passive into active voice

Revising passive voice into active voice helps improve your writing. Why?

IT SOUNDS MORE NATURAL

More than any other technique, using active voice and specifying who performs an action changes the character of your writing.[11] Active voice sounds direct and vigorous. A reader understands a sentence in active voice more quickly and easily, since it reflects how the human mind naturally thinks and processes information.[12] For example, saying, "We recruited patients and clinicians," sounds stronger and more specific than "Patients and clinicians were recruited."

IT SAVES WORDS

An active sentence often saves words; a passive sentence often uses more words. A whole document that uses just passive sentences can be 30% longer than one that just uses active sentences.[13]

IT AVOIDS THE *WHO-DONE-IT* MYSTERY

In addition to being shorter and more direct, an active sentence forces you to name the *actor* or causal agent of your narrative. With a passive sentence, the *actor* tends to go unnamed.[14] There is a deep human instinct to find cause-and-effect relationships. We naturally ask, *what causes something to happen*? The literary genre of the *who-done-it* mystery plays upon this instinct. Passive voice often obscures the *actor*; this can send the reader on a mental wild goose chase trying to solve the mystery of *who-done-it*. Writing in active voice and naming the *actor* avoids this problem.

Exercise 4.B. Revise passive into active voice
For each sentence:

1. Read it out loud and underline the <u>subject once</u> and the <u>verb twice</u>. Draw braces around any {past participle}. Count the number of words in the sentence.
2. Is the sentence active, passive or neither?
3. Revise each passive sentence to put it in active voice, making any other changes you can think of to improve reading ease. Count the number of words in your revision.

Compare your answers to the Exercise Key in Appendix 3.

> **1. Daily 24-hour urine collections for volume and urinary sodium excretion were performed for 72 hours.[15]**
>
> **2. COPD can be classified with respect to both phenotype and disease severity.[16]**

Note: *COPD* stands for *chronic obstructive pulmonary disease.*

> **3. Once a drug is administered, it is absorbed and distributed to its site of action, where it interacts with targets (such as receptors and enzymes), undergoes metabolism, and is then excreted.[17]**
>
> **4. Researchers have found evidence for bias related to specific design features of primary studies of diagnostic studies.[18]**
>
> **5. The incidence of major injury in each of the cohorts was calculated per 10,000 person-years.[19]**
>
> **6. The exact pathophysiologic mechanism for scoliosis is unknown.[20]**

C. When should you use passive voice?

Use passive voice sparingly and purposefully.[21] Passive voice has proper uses.[22] It can help keep the same or similar subjects in a series of sentences, thus making for better flow and easier reading. For example, in the following journal excerpt, the last sentence is in passive voice. This helps keep the narrative focused on the study population.

We conducted a nested case-control study within the Kaiser Permanente Northern California (KPNC) integrated health-care system, which provides comprehensive inpatient and outpatient services for approximately 3.3 million members. The KPNC membership approximates the underlying census race/ethnicity and socioeconomic distributions of the Northern California region. Prescription drug benefits are utilized by more than 90% of members.[23] *(WSEG = 56/18.6/0.0/19.0)*

Passive voice can help move a word to a strategic part of the sentence to give emphasis or to connect to a word in the preceding sentence. For example, Shakespeare uses this technique in the opening line of his play, *Richard III*: "Now is the winter of our discontent, made glorious summer by this sun of York."

Passive voice can also help where the *action* is important, but the *agent* is not. For example, the following excerpt defines "vitamin B$_{12}$ deficiency" without telling who came up with this definition.

Vitamin B$_{12}$ deficiency was defined as the presence of 1 of the following: the first diagnostic code for vitamin B$_{12}$ deficiency, using *International Classification of Diseases, Ninth Revision* codes 281.0 (pernicious anemia), 281.1 (other vitamin B$_{12}$ deficiency anemia), 266.2 (specified at KPNC as vitamin B$_{12}$ deficiency), or specific text diagnoses of vitamin B$_{12}$ deficiency in the problem list; an abnormally low value of serum vitamin B$_{12}$; or a new and at least 6-month supply of injectable vitamin B$_{12}$ supplements.[24] (Italics in original.) *(WSEG = 80/80.0/0.0/20.9)*

In this regard, passive voice can sometimes save words, as in a list of procedures, where one item is manipulated in several different ways.[25]

SUMMARY

Use passive voice, sparingly, when you have a good reason. Otherwise, use active.

D. Minimize forms of *to be* and *to have*

If you want to write vividly, search for the verbs *to be* and *to have* and revise to minimize them. Sometimes you need them, and sometimes you don't. If you don't need them, try to avoid them as main verbs.[26] (Other forms of the verb *to be* include *be, am, is, are, was, were, have been, will be,* etc. Other forms of the verb *to have* include *have, had, have had, had had, will have, will have had,* etc.)

To be and *to have* often appear in a sentence that lacks action. (In this case, they are called *intransitive* verbs, since the subject of the sentence neither acts

Table 4-2. **A vivid sentence describes action**

No action (intransitive verb)	Action (transitive verb)
Smoking status <u>was</u> {categorized} as current, past, or never smoked.[i] (*WSEG = 10/10.0/52.8/8.3*)	<u>We noted</u> for each patient whether they: smoke now, used to smoke, or never smoked. (*WSEG = 15/15.0/84.4/5.2*)
Although <u>it can be</u> transient, <u>older persons **are**</u> more likely to have persistent tinnitus.[ii] (*WSEG = 16/16.0/ 16.1/14.9*)	An older patient <u>tends</u> to get persistent tinnitus more often, though <u>it</u> sometimes <u>lasts</u> only a short while. (*WSEG = 18/18.0/ 56.9/9.7*)
The illness episode <u>was</u> {classified} as VCD if <u>any test was</u> positive.[iii] (*WSEG = 12/12.0/53.6/8.7*)	<u>We counted</u> an illness episode as VCD, if the blood <u>tested</u> positive. (*WSEG = 12/12.0/ 60.7/7.7*)

Note: VCD stands for *virologically confirmed dengue.*
[i]Aakre, "Postoperative Acute Respiratory Distress," *Mayo Clinic Proc* 183 (see chap. 1, n. 19).
[ii]Yew K, "Diagnostic Approach to Patients with Tinnitus," *Am Fam Phys* 89, no. 2 (2014): 106.
[iii]Villar L, et al. "Efficacy of a Tetravalent Dengue," *N Eng J Med* 372 (2015), under "Procedures," http://www.nemj.org/doi/full/10.1056/NEJMoa1411037?query=TOC.

upon anything else, nor receives action.) Instead, they describe a state of being or a state of possession. By contrast, a sentence that describes action sounds more vivid. Table 4-2 shows examples of sentences we revised in active voice to show action.

For each example in Table 4-2, the sentence on the left contains a form of the verb *to be* (*was, be* or *are*). It sounds less vigorous than the revision on the right, which uses a verb in active voice to describe action.

You also need to use a form of the verb, *to have* to write in the perfect tense; but the simple past tense, which does not use *have*, often serves just as well. See Table 4-3.

Table 4-3. **Revising to eliminate *to have***

Perfect tense using **have**	Simple past tense without **have**
No recent studies <u>have</u> evaluated methylphenidate in the treatment of fatigue in general palliative care settings.[i] (*WSEG = 16/16.0/16.1/14.9*)	<u>We found</u> no recent study on the use of methylphenidate to treat fatigue in a general palliative care setting. (*WSEG = 19/19.0/45.0/11.6*)

[i]Onishi E, Biagioli F, Safranek S, "Methylphenidate for Management of Fatigue in the Palliative Care Setting," *Am Fam Phys* 89, no. 2 (2014): 124.

SUMMARY

If you want to write vividly, look for sentences that use a form of *to be* or *to have*, and try to re-write them in active voice using a verb that shows action.

Exercise 4.D. Minimize forms of to be *or* to have
For each sentence:

1. Read it out loud. Underline each form of the verb *to be* or *to have*. Draw braces around any {past participle}.
2. Revise to eliminate any form of *to be* or *to have*, and instead, use a verb in active voice. Make any other changes you can think of to improve reading ease.

Compare your answers to the Exercise Key in Appendix 3.

1. A linear regression was used to assess all trends over time.[27]

2. Such assessment is not a straightforward addition of reported causes. Because there are likely to be many more data reported for levels of all-cause mortality than there are for individual causes, the independent assessment of age-specific mortality is crucial to constrain the often less robust estimates of cause-specific mortality within each population group defined by age and sex.[28]

3. The current hospitalist-ambulist division of general medical care has made important contributions to patient care, but it leaves much to be desired, especially with regard to personalization and continuity of care.[29]

4. Although they are part of a randomized trial, the participants represent a selected group of people who have chosen to participate and who attended the follow-up.[30]

5. Inhaled corticosteroids (ICSs) have had a central role in the management of asthma, even before publication of the first *Guidelines for the Diagnosis and Management of Asthma* in 1991.[31]

6. The cremasteric reflex, which is elicited by pinching the medial thigh, causes elevation of the testicle.[32]

E. Identify nominalization

One of the over-used writing habits that make medical writing hard to read is *nominalization. Nominalization* is the process of making an abstract noun out of a verb or adjective. (What is an *abstract* noun? It is a noun that relates to the world of ideas, often something we can't touch or see. By contrast, a *red rubber ball* is a real-world, concrete object, since you can touch and see it. We'll talk more

Table 4-4. **Examples of nominalization**

Verb becomes an abstract noun			Adjective becomes an abstract noun		
isolate	=>	isolation	careless	=>	carelessness
expose	=>	exposure	competent	=>	competency
complicate	=>	complication	orderly	=>	orderliness
investigate	=>	investigation	clean	=>	cleanliness
approve	=>	approval	sufficient	=>	sufficiency
limit	=>	limitation	effective	=>	effectiveness
recommend	=>	recommendation	effective	=>	efficacy
replace	=>	replacement	sensitive	=>	sensitivity
inform	=>	information	normal	=>	normalization
negate	=>	negative	negative	=>	negativity

about *abstract* and *concrete* in the next chapter.) Table 4-4 shows examples of nominalization.

A nominalized verb tends to make for a long, abstract word. Because the word is long, it can drive down the reading ease score. Because the word is abstract, it tends to make the writing less vivid.

WHEN SHOULD YOU USE A NOMINALIZATION?

There are a few situations where nominalization helps you present good science clearly and concisely. The first is where the nominalization refers to a name, fixed expression, or well-known subject. Examples:

- Few problems so divide Americans as *abortion* on demand.
- The Equal Rights *Amendment* surfaced as an issue in past elections.[33]

The second is where the nominalization serves as a short subject that refers to a previous sentence, and promotes a smooth flow of logic. Table 4-5 gives a few examples of this.

Table 4-5. **Using nominalization as a short subject to promote the smooth flow of logic**

Instead of	With nominalization
The hospital administrator accepted *what the doctor requested.*	The hospital administrator accepted *the doctor's request.*
All *these things they argue* depend upon an unproven claim.	*These arguments* all depend upon an unproven claim.

SUMMARY

Use nominalization when you have a good reason; otherwise, avoid it.

Exercise 4.E. Identify nominalization
For each sentence, read it out loud and underline each instance of <u>nominalization</u>.
Compare your answers to the Exercise Key in Appendix 3.

1. To curb such empirical use, a report from the Infectious Diseases Society of America (IDSA) is calling for steps to boost the development of better diagnostic tests, to reduce regulatory hurdles for new tests, and to improve clinical use of infectious disease diagnostics.[34]

2. In sub-Saharan Africa and southeast Asia, peer or community counselling and condom distribution among female sex workers was estimated to be cost effective, at US$86 per infection averted and $5 per DALY averted (all costs from here expressed in 2012 US$), and was more cost-effective than school-based education, voluntary counselling and testing, prevention of mother-to-child transmissions, and STI treatment.[35]

Note: *DALY* stands for *disability adjusted life year. STI* stands for *sexually transmitted infection.*

3. We hypothesized that the administration of fixed-duration antibiotic therapy (4 days) after source control would lead to equivalent outcomes and a shorter duration of therapy as compared with the traditional strategy of administration of antibiotics until 2 days after the resolution of the physiological abnormalities related to SIRS.[36]

Note: *SIRS* stands for *systemic inflammatory response syndrome.*

4. Over 93% of participants in the control arm aged 40-49 returned their annual questionnaire, whereas compliance with annual breast examination screening for those in the control arm aged 50-59 varied between 89% (for screen 2) and 85% (for screen 5); only questionnaires were obtained for 3% to 7% of the women.[37]

5. For many of these reasons, evidence-based reviews generally make authoritative statements on the degree of evidence in support of the use of each medication for a defined disorder, but they are not always conducive to the development of practical algorithms for the management of disorders of varying severity and a lengthy natural history.[38]

6. If history or examination findings raise concern for intracranial lesions, magnetic resonance imaging of the brain can be useful for further evaluation, with particular scrutiny of the skull base.[39]

Table 4-6. **Minimize nominalization to improve vividness**

Nominalized verbs	*Revised to reduce nominalization*
The factors that can affect patient outcome include complete macro- and microscopic tumor <u>resection</u> (R0-resection), the depth of tumor <u>infiltration</u> (T-category), the <u>presence</u> of lymph node <u>metastasis</u> (N-category), and the <u>presence</u> or <u>absence</u> of lymphatic vessel <u>invasion (L VI)</u>.[i] (*WSEG= 39/39.0/6.7/22.0*)	Many factors affect patient outcome, including: 1. how much of the tumor is removed (R0-resection), 2. how deep the tumor infiltrates (T-category), 3. whether the cancer metastasizes to the lymph nodes (N-category), or 4. whether it gets into the lymph vessels (L VI). (*WSEG= 39/39.0/94.3/2.3*)

[i]Brücher B, M Kitajima, and J Siewert, "Undervalued Criteria in the Evaluation of Multimodal Trials for Upper GI Cancers," *Cancer Invest* 32, no. 10 (2014), under "Multimodal Therapy," http://www.ncbi.nlm.nih.gov/pmc/articles/PMC4266078.

F. Convert nominalization into a verb in active voice

You can often improve reading ease and make your writing more vivid by avoiding nominalization. Since nominalization is a grammatical form, unless it is part of a name or a fixed expression, a nominalized term is rarely an essential scientific term.

The example in Table 4-6 uses many nominalizations. None of these nominalizations is an essential scientific term, since we can replace each one with a verb in root form, or by substituting a plain-English equivalent.

SUMMARY

Avoid nominalization unless you can give a reason why it helps you write clearly and concisely.

Exercise 4.F. Convert nominalization into a verb in active voice
For each sentence:

1. Read it out loud and underline each <u>nominalization</u>.
2. Revise to convert the nominalization to a verb in active voice. Make any other changes you can think of to improve reading ease.

Compare your answers to the Exercise Key in Appendix 3.

1. Data from each trial were entered on an intention-to-treat basis according to the recommendations of the Cochrane Collaboration

and the Preferred Reporting Items for Systematic Reviews and Meta-analyses (PRISMA) statement.[40]

2. Accurate estimation of the number of deaths in each age and sex group in a country, region, or worldwide is a crucial starting point for assessment of the global burden of disease.[41]

3. For some drugs, however, oxidation leads to conversion of a pro-drug into an active compound.[42]

4. After five years of counselling a significant effect on lifestyle was seen, with a substantial reduction in the prevalence of smoking, improved dietary habits, sustained physical activity (among men), and a decrease in binge drinking.[43]

5. Much evidence has been amassed in support of asthma treatment with ICSs.[44]

Note: *ICSs* stands for *inhaled corticosteroids*.

6. In its 2011 recommendation statement, the U.S. Preventative Services Task Force did not find sufficient evidence for or against screening for bladder cancer in asymptomatic adults[45]

Conclusion

If you want to write vividly, *prefer active voice*. When you can, revise passive into active, minimize *to be* and *to have*, and convert nominalization into a verb in active voice.

In the next chapter, we discuss the difference between *concrete* and *abstract*.

Notes

1. Williams, *Style: Lessons in Clarity*, 71 (see Preface, n. 8).
2. Strunk W, White E B, *The Elements of Style* (New York: Macmillan, 1979), 18–19.
3. Greene, *Writing Science in Plain*, 22–28 (see Preface, n. 7).
4. Plain Language Action and Information Network, *Federal Plain Language Guidelines* (March 2011, Revised May 2011), 20–21, available at www.plainlanguage.gov.
5. Martinez-Garcia, "Effect of CPAP on," 2409 (see chap. 3, n. 8).
6. Beyrer C, et al., "An Action Agenda for HIV and Sex Workers," *Lancet* 385, no. 9964 (January 2015), under "Introduction," http://www.thelancet.com/journals/lancet/article/PIIS0140-6736(14)60933-8/fulltext.
7. Furie, "Do Pharmacogenetics Have a," 2345 (see chap. 2, n. 30).
8. Feeney, "Antiviral Treatment of Hepatitis," under "HCV Life Cycle and Natural Course," (see chap. 3, n. 5).
9. Iyer V, Lim K, "Chronic Cough: An Update," *Mayo Clinic Proc* 88, no. 10 (2013): 1116.
10. Tsang K, Hartmark-Hill J, "Ticagrelor (Brilinta) for Secondary Prevention of Thrombotic Events Following Acute Coronary Syndrome," *Am Fam Phys* 88, no. 12 (2013): 822.

11. Plain Language Action and Information Network, *Federal Plain Language Guidelines*, 20 (see chap. 4, n. 4).
12. Office of Investor Education and Assistance, *A Plain English Handbook* (Washington DC: US Securities and Exchange Commission, August 1998), 21.
13. Greene, *Writing Science in Plain*, 22–23 (see Preface, n. 7).
14. Ibid.
15. Chen H, et al. "Low-Dose Dopamine or Low-Dose Nesiritide in Acute Heart Failure with Renal Dysfunction: The ROSE Acute Heart Failure Randomized Trial," *JAMA* 310, no. 23 (2013): 2534.
16. Mannino, "Global Burden of COPD," 766 (see chap. 1, n. 8).
17. Weinshilbourn, "Inheritance and Drug Response," 529 (see chap. 1, n. 17).
18. Mallett, "Systematic Reviews of Diagnostic," under "Introduction" (see chap. 1, n. 18).
19. Lai M, et al. "Long-Term Use of Zolpidem Increases the Risk of Major Injury: A Population-Based Cohort Study," *Mayo Clinic Proc* 89, no. 5 (2014): 590.
20. Horne, "Adolescent Idiopathic Scoliosis: Diagnosis," 193 (see chap. 1, n. 12).
21. Office of Investor Education and Assistance, *A Plain English Handbook*, 19 (see chap. 4, n. 12).
22. Wydick, *Plain English for Lawyers*, 31–32 (see Intro, n. 8).
23. Lam J, et al. "Proton Pump Inhibitor and Histamine 2 Receptor Antagonist Use and Vitamin B$_{12}$ Deficiency," *JAMA* 310, no. 22 (2013): 2436.
24. Ibid.
25. Greene, *Writing Science in Plain*, 22–28 (see Preface, n. 7).
26. Ibid.
27. Kawwass J, et al. "Trends and Outcomes for Donors Oocyte Cycles in the United States, 2000–2010," *JAMA* 310, no. 22 (2013): 2427.
28. Wang, "Age-specific and Sex-specific Mortality," 2072 (see chap. 1, n. 24).
29. Goroll A, Hunt D, "Bridging the Hospitalist-Primary Care Divide through Collaborative Care," *N Eng J Med* 372, no. 4 (2015), http://www.nejm.org/doi/full/10.1056/NEJMp1411416.
30. Jorgensen, "Effect of Screening and," under "Introduction," (see chap. 1, n. 10).
31. Scanlon P, "Pneumonia Associated with Inhaled Corticosteroid Use in Chronic Obstructive Pulmonary Disease: Another Perspective," *Mayo Clinic Proc* 89, no. 2 (2014): 139.
32. Sharp V, Kieran K, Arlen A, "Testicular Torsion: Diagnosis, Evaluation and Management," *Am Fam Phys* 88, no. 12 (2013): 836.
33. Williams, *Style: Lessons in Clarity*, 48–49 (see Preface, n. 8).
34. Kuehn B, "IDSA: Better, Faster Diagnostics for Infectious Diseases Needed to Curb Overtreatment, Antibiotic Resistance," *JAMA* 310, no. 22 (2013): 2385.
35. Beyrer, "An Action Agenda for," under "Costing of a New Response" (see chap. 4, n. 6).
36. Sawyer R, et al. "Trial of Short-Course Antimicrobial Therapy for Intraabdominal Infection," *N Eng J Med* 372, no. 21 (2015): 1997.
37. Miller, "Twenty Five Year Follow-up," under "Methods" (see chap. 2, n. 20).
38. Silber, "Willis-Ekbom Disease Foundation," 978 (see chap. 3, n. 12).
39. Malaty J, Malaty I, "Smell and Taste Disorders in Primary Care," *Am Fam Phys* 88, no. 12 (2013): 854.
40. Udell J, et al. "Associated Between Influenza Vaccination and Cardiovascular Outcomes in High-Risk Patients: A Meta-Analysis," *JAMA* 310, no. 16 (2013): 1712.
41. Wang, "Age-specific and Sex-specific Mortality," 2071 (see chap. 1, n. 24).
42. Caraco, "Genes and the Response," 2868 (see chap. 2, n. 43).
43. Jorgensen, "Effect of Screening and," under "Introduction" (see chap. 1, n. 10).
44. Scanlon, "Pneumonia Associated with Inhaled," 139 (see chap. 4, n. 31).
45. Sharp, "Assessment of Asymptomatic Microscopic," 747 (see chap. 1, n. 28).

CHAPTER 5

Prefer concrete language

Few people have the imagination for reality.—Johann Wolfgang von Goethe

The practice of medicine deals with both the real world and the world of abstract ideas, but traditional medical writing tends to be overly abstract. This chapter presents tips for making your writing more vivid by preferring concrete language. Making writing more vivid often goes hand-in-hand with improving reading ease. The first step is to learn to tell the difference between *abstract* and *concrete* language.

A. Identify abstract and concrete subjects

What do we mean by *abstract* and *concrete*? A *concrete* object is something from the real world, like a doctor, a patient or a test tube. A doctor performs many real-world actions, such as looking in a patient's ear or throat, listening to their heart, or making an incision.

By contrast, an *abstract* idea is "a theoretical way of looking at things; something that exists only in idealized form."[1] Abstract ideas include concepts, theories, calculations and procedures. A medical diagnosis is abstract, since it involves developing a theory of the nature and cause of a condition based on analyzing a patient's signs, symptoms and test results.

One of the best-known sentences in the English language is the Pledge of Allegiance of the United States. "I pledge allegiance to the Flag of the United States of America, and to the Republic for which it stands, one Nation under God, indivisible, with liberty and justice for all."

In this pledge, the *Flag* is a concrete, real-world object you can see and touch. The sentence also deals with some abstract ideas: *the United States of America, the Republic, the Nation, indivisible, liberty* and *justice*. These ideas are important, but hard to visualize. The pledge presents the flag as a vivid, colorful symbol to represent these ideas.

It's not always easy to make a clear distinction between abstract and concrete. For example, if you turn on a water tap, you can see whether the water runs fast or slowly; this is a real-world observation. If you measure the amount of water that flows within a particular time, you can compute the rate of flow; this is an abstract calculation. (You might say, merely observing that the water is running fast or slowly involves abstract thinking).

Table 5-1 gives examples of medical terms that describe the real world and the world of abstract ideas.

Table 5-1. **Examples of real-world and abstract medical terms**

Real world	*World of abstract ideas*
heart	cardiac
blood	blood type
balance	hydrostatic equilibrium
heartbeat, rhythm, stethoscope	pulse, heart rate
pump, flow	circulate, blood pressure, arrhythmia
vein, artery, arteriole	circulation, circulatory system, coronary output
scalpel, cut, incision	surgical procedure
pill, tablet, shot, injection, IV bolus	dose, dosage, dosing, dosing regimen
tumor, cancer cell	lymphoma (diagnosis)
"zapping" a tumor	treatment, protocol, therapy
die, death	mortality
mouth, throat, stomach, gut, small intestine, large intestine	digestion, digestive system
lung, breath, breathing	pulmonary, respiration, respiratory system
cough (symptom)	cold (diagnosis)
lymph node	lymphatic system
nerve, spinal cord	nervous system
sperm, egg, ovary, womb, testicle, embryo	reproductive system, embryology, ovulation
vertebrae, spine, bone, skeleton	skeletal system
warm, hot, thermometer	fever, temperature
pee, urine	urinary tract, urinary output
biopsy	pathology, pathological analysis
computer, calculator, ruler	statistical analysis, standard deviation, mean, median, mode, average, error, measurement

SUMMARY

It's important to develop a good sense of whether a word or phrase sounds abstract or concrete. If you favor concrete language, it will help make your writing more vivid.

Exercise 5.A. Identify whether a subject is abstract or concrete
For each sentence:

1. Read the sentence out loud. Underline the <u>subject</u>.
2. Is the subject abstract or concrete?

Compare your answers to the Exercise Key in Appendix 3.

> **1. Strengths of this study include the relatively large sample size, the prospective assessment of leukocyte telomere length with blood samples collected prior to HCT and the availability of detailed covariate data known to influence transplant outcome.**[2]

Note: *HCT* stands for *hematopoietic cell transplant.*

> **2. Fourth, individuals with similar smoking and exposure histories can vary a great deal in the severity of their disease and response to intervention.**[3]

> **3. Vitamin K plays a single role in human biology—as a cofactor for the synthesis of γ-carboxyglutamic acid.**[4]

> **4. Previous research on systematic reviews of diagnostic tests noted poor methods and reporting.**[5]

> **5. We defined AMI by the presence of an increase and/or decrease of cardiac biomarkers (preferably troponin) with at least 1 value above the 99th percentile of the upper reference limit together with evidence of myocardial ischemia with at least 1 of the following: (1) symptoms of ischemia, (2) electrocardiographic changes indicative of new ischemia (new ST-T changes or new left bundle branch block), (3) pathological Q waves on the electrocardiogram, and (4) imaging evidence of new loss of viable myocardium or new regional wall motion abnormality.**[6]

Note: *AMI* stands for *acute myocardial infarction.*

> **6. Documentation of the history, physical examination, diagnostic study results, clinical impression, and diagnostic reasoning is vital not only for medical care, but also for legal purposes.**[7]

B. Revise abstract into concrete

With medical writing, sometimes you need to talk about a real-world object (e.g., a patient, a cancer cell, or a placenta). Sometimes you need to talk about a real-world event (e.g., a patient dies, bleeds, vomits). Sometimes you need to talk about an abstract idea (e.g., a cause and effect relationship, a diagnosis, a process). No matter what you're writing about, you often have a choice about how you frame the discussion. Using concrete language tends to make your writing more vivid and memorable. It also favors shorter words and better reading ease scores.

One strategy for writing clearly and concisely is to make a sentence's subject a concrete noun rather than an abstract noun. Let's consider an example:

> Because of the estrogen-mediated increase in thyroid-binding globulin, the increased volume of the distribution of the thyroid hormone, and the placental metabolism and transport of maternal thyroxine, there is a 20% to 40% increase in the thyroid hormone requirement as early as the fourth week of gestation.[8] *(WSEG = 47/47.0/0.7/24.8)*

This sentence uses an abstract subject, *there*, which lays buried deep within the long sentence.

We can do a few things to simplify this sentence. We can use a concrete subject, *woman*. We can put her at the start of the sentence. We can split the sentence into shorter pieces. "A woman needs 20% to 40% more thyroid hormone by her 4th week of pregnancy. Why? Because her estrogen causes an increase in thyroid-binding globulin. This thyroid hormone spreads over an increased volume of distribution. The placenta metabolizes and uses some of the mother's thyroxine." *(WSEG = 45/9.0/47.3/8.8)*. With these changes, the main subject and verb make natural points of interest that make the science more vivid and improve reading ease.

Exercise 5.B. Revise abstract into concrete
For each sentence:

1. Read it out loud and underline the <u>subject</u>.
2. Revise to use a concrete subject and replace other abstract language with concrete language. Make any other changes you can think of to improve reading ease.

Compare your answers to the Exercise Key in Appendix 3.

> **1. During the past several decades, mean maternal age at delivery of a first infant has increased steadily to 25.2 years in the United States and 30 years in Germany and Britain in 2009.[9]**

2. **Fifth, the airflow limitation or obstruction that happens in COPD is caused by a mixture of small airway disease, parenchymal destruction (emphysema), and, in many cases, increased airways responsiveness (asthma).**[10]

3. **The goal of therapy is to keep the INR in the therapeutic range, since patients with an INR that is subtherapeutic are at increased risk for thrombosis and patients with an INR that is supratherapeutic are at increased risk for bleeding.**[11]

Note: *INR* stands for *international normalized ratio*.

4. **Ischaemic heart disease remains a leading cause of morbidity and mortality worldwide.**[12]

5. **Antihypertensive medication use was retrieved from the internal pharmacy-dispensing records.**[13]

6. **Over the past 75 years, the number of U.S. women receiving prenatal care has steadily increased.**[14]

C. Use nouns and verbs to carry the weight of meaning

Write using nouns and verbs, not with adjectives and adverbs.—Strunk and White[15]

Adjectives and adverbs can add important detail to a sentence, but use them sparingly. Studies show that articles in other fields tend to use between 11% and 18% adjectives and adverbs.[16] When your writing exceeds this "normal" range, consider cutting adjectives and adverbs and revise to focus more on nouns and verbs. This helps make your writing more clear and vivid.

What makes a sentence clear? One thing is, the reader can quickly grasp how each word relates to the others. Consider a short sentence that uses only nouns and verbs: "Jane threw Dick the ball." *(WSEG = 5/5/100.0/0.0).* Since this sentence uses just three nouns and one verb, the reader easily sees how each word relates to the others.

- *Jane* (the subject) did the throwing
- *threw* (the verb) is what Jane did with the ball
- *the ball* (the direct object) is what Jane threw to Dick
- *Dick* (the indirect object) is the one to whom Jane threw the ball

Adding a few short adjectives provides vivid detail but hardly changes the reading ease score: "Jane threw Dick the red rubber ball." *(WSEG = 7/7.0/100.0/0.6).* As we add more adjectives and adverbs, we start to make the sentence more subtle, interesting and complex. But we also start to cloud the relationship between words: "Pregnant Jane impulsively threw the half-inflated red rubber ball to an equally astonished Dick." *(wseg = 14/14.0/35.5/11.7)*.

FAVOR REAL-WORLD ADJECTIVES OVER ABSTRACT ONES

Not all adjectives and adverbs are created equal. The real-world adjectives *red* and *rubber* are short and simple. They give vivid details about the physical properties of the ball and may help the reader to visualize it. On the other hand, *impulsively* and *astonished* are longer, abstract words. They represent Jane and Dick's states of mind as Jane throws the ball, which may be hard to visualize. It takes more mental effort for a reader to process these abstract ideas.

Jane's pregnancy adds a further complication. Of course, pregnancy is a real-world condition. Depending on how far along she is, Jane's pregnancy may seem like more of a physical state—easy to visualize—or a state of mind. This sentence also implies a question, Is Jane's impulsive behavior related to her pregnancy? A novelist may choose to write this way to make the story more interesting, but a medical author usually just wants to explain the science clearly.

SUMMARY

Adjectives and adverbs can add important detail, but they also complicate. It takes skill to manage this tradeoff and decide: *What information is important?* and *How much can I pack into one sentence?* Overusing adjectives and adverbs—especially abstract ones—can sap vitality from a sentence. Cutting down on adjectives and adverbs is one way to make your writing more vivid. Adjectives and adverbs that relate to physical properties often help make your sentence more vivid; those that relate to abstract ideas may have the opposite effect.

Exercise 5.C. Use nouns and verbs to carry the weight of meaning
For each sentence:

1. Read it out loud and underline each <u>adjective</u> and <u>adverb</u>. Count the number of words you underlined. Compute adjectives and adverbs as a percentage of total words.
2. Revise to reduce the number of adjectives and adverbs. Make any other changes you can think of to improve reading ease. Compute a new percentage of adjectives and adverbs.

Compare your answers to the Exercise Key in Appendix 3.

1. But the physician's subsequent choice to designate the hospital discharge as against medical advice and pursue the formalized process

associated with it (eg, specialized discharge forms) has no evidence-based utility for patient care, is not legally required, and has been shown to be associated with a reduced willingness for the patient to return for future care.[17]

2. We used these advances, and a further extension of the Brass relational model life tables, to develop a time series of annual age-specific mortality rates for 187 countries from 1970 to 2010, including uncertainty.[18]

3. The bimodal distribution of plasma isoniazid concentrations in subjects with genetically determined fast or slow rates of acetylation in one of those early studies strikingly illustrates the consequences of inherited variations in this pathway for drug metabolism (Fig. 2).[19]

4. There was evidence of bias when primary studies did not provide an adequate description of either the diagnostic (index) test or the patients, when different reference tests were used for positive and negative index tests, or when a case-control design was used.[20]

5. The use of nonergot dopamine agonists has become widespread, but increasing experience with these drugs has revealed treatment-limiting adverse effects, including the development of augmentation and impulse control disorders.[21]

6. Support groups could be helpful with diet maintenance.[22]

D. Write in the singular

One simple way to make your writing more vivid is to write in the singular.[23] This can also help boost your reading ease score. One thing that makes writing abstract and hard to visualize is a big number. It's easy to imagine one thing. It's a little harder to think of two or three. It's harder still to imagine a dozen or a hundred.

You can easily imagine one puppy. It's harder to imagine a mother dog nursing a litter of puppies. You probably can't imagine 101 Dalmatians, as in the children's novel by Dodie Smith.[24] For us, as in the novel, 101 is a math calculation. It's an overwhelming number of dogs, not something you can easily imagine.

If you write in the singular, you won't be able to use the plural to avoid the awkward *he or she, as the case may be.* The alternative we use is the singular pronoun, *they,* which has historical precedent and seems to be gaining ground.[25]

Let's consider examples of how writing in the singular can help make your writing more vivid. See Table 5-2. For each example, we took a sentence with a plural subject, revised it to make the subject singular, and then, made other changes to improve reading ease.

Table 5-2. **Revising to use a singular subject**

Plural subject	Singular subject	Other changes
<u>Patients</u> with symptoms suggestive of acute myocardial infarction (AMI) account for approximately 10% of all emergency department (ED) consultations.[i] *(WSEG = 19/19.0/0.0/19.1)*	<u>The patient</u> with symptoms suggestive of acute myocardial infarction (AMI) accounts for approximately 10% of all emergency department (ED) consultations. *(WSEG = 19/19.0/0.0/18.7)*	<u>The patient</u> with symptoms that suggest acute myocardial infarction (AMI) accounts for 1 in 10 ER visits. *(WSEG = 17/17.0/40.2/ 11.8)*
<u>Patients</u> want and expect to have a well-rested and competent surgeon performing <u>their</u> operations.[ii] *(WSEG = 14/ 14.0/29.4/12.6)*	<u>A patient</u> wants and expects to have a well-rested and competent surgeon performing <u>their</u> operation. *(WSEG = 15/ 15.0/33.6/12.2)*	<u>A patient</u> expects <u>their</u> surgeon to be competent and well-rested when they operate on <u>them</u>. *(WSEG = 16/16.0/58.4/9.0)*

[i]Reichlin T, et al. "One-Hour Rule-Out and Rule-In of Acute Myocardial Infarction Using High-Sensitivity Cardiac Troponin T," *Arch Intern Med* 172, no. 16 (2012), under "Conclusions," http://archinte.jamanetwork.com/article.aspx?articleid=1309579.
[ii]Zinner, "Surgeons, Sleep and Patient," 1808 (see chap. 2, n. 28).

SUMMARY

Writing in the singular is an easy way to write more vividly and improve reading ease.

Exercise 5.D. Write in the singular
For each sentence:

1. Read it out loud and underline each element that makes something plural.
2. Where you can, revise to put the sentence in the singular. Make any other changes you can think of to improve reading ease.

Compare your answers to the Exercise Key in Appendix 3.

   1. All patients had a telephone assessment of vital status and rehospitalization at 60 and 180 days from randomization.[26]

   2. All these hypotheses probably have elements of truth since COPD is a classic gene-by-environment disease with various manifestations that include increased airways reactivity, a characteristic response to infections, abnormal cellular repair, and development of complications or comorbid disorders.[27]

3. After the intake of identical doses of a given agent, some patients may have clinically significant adverse effects, whereas others may have no therapeutic response.[28]

4. Participants were referred to their general practitioner for medical treatment, if relevant.[29]

5. All patients had angiographically defined CAD with at least 1 vessel that met the American College of Cardiology/American Heart Association (AHA/ACC) class I or II indications for PCI, and only those who received implants with drug-eluting stents were considered eligible for the study.[30]

Note: *CAD* stands for *coronary artery disease*. *PCI* stands for *percutaneous coronary intervention*.

6. Tinnitus occurs in most persons with normal hearing who are exposed to silence.[31]

E. Talk in terms of one doctor treating one patient

The goal of medicine is one human life at a time—to keep one patient healthy—to heal one patient—to keep one patient alive—to relieve one patient's suffering. No matter what they do now, every doctor has seen a patient in an exam room and can imagine this scene vividly.

Regrettably, traditional medical writing often adopts a needlessly abstract way of talking about multiple patients, patient populations, or a disease with no patient at all. Even where a study deals with a group of patients or multiple patient populations, you can often frame the discussion in terms of one doctor treating one patient.

The fields of genetics, pharmacology, epidemiology, and statistics deal with complex problems that affect millions of lives. These problems are solved through abstract thought. Still, framing an issue in terms of how it affects one patient often brings it into sharper focus.

Let's consider some examples in Table 5-3. For each example, we start with a sentence that deals with multiple patients or no patient. We underlined the subject once and the verb twice. Then we revised to talk about one patient. Then we made other changes to improve reading ease.

Exercise 5.E. Talk in terms of one doctor treating one patient
For each sentence:
1. Read it out loud.
2. Revise to talk about one doctor treating one patient. Make any other changes you can think of to improve reading ease.

Table 5-3. **Revising to talk about one patient**

Multiple patients/no patient	One patient	Other changes
All children **were scheduled** for visits at months 0, 6, and 12 for vaccination and at month 13 for follow-up blood sampling.[i] *(WSEG = 22/22.0/57.6/10.6)*	Each child <u>was scheduled</u> for a visit at months 0, 6 and 12 for vaccination and at month 13 for a follow-up blood sample. *(WSEG = 24/24.0/62.6/10.4)*	We <u>scheduled</u> each child to get the vaccine at months 0, 6 and 12 with a follow-up blood sample at month 13. *(WSEG = 22/22.0/ 69.1/9.0)*
For example, several studies <u>have used</u> common genetic variants near the gene encoding C-reactive protein (CRP) to show that raised high-sensitivity CRP is unlikely to affect the risk of heart disease causally.[ii] *(WSEG = 32/32.0/23.6/17.9)*	For example, several studies <u>have used</u> common genetic variants near the gene encoding C-reactive protein (CRP) to show that, if a patient has a raised high-sensitivity CRP, it is unlikely to affect their risk of heart disease. *(WSEG = 37/37.0/29.8/18.2)*	If a <u>patient has</u> a raised high-sensitivity C-reactive protein (CRP), does it affect their risk of heart disease? Many studies have looked at common gene variants near the gene coding CRP, and it seems the answer is, *no.* *(WSEG = 38/19.0/65.1/8.8)*

[i]Villar, "Efficacy of a Tetravalent," under "Procedures," (see chap. 4, Table 4-2).

[ii]Frayling T, "Statins and Type 2 Diabetes: Genetic Studies on Target," *Lancet* 385 (2015): 311.

Compare your answers to the Exercise Key in Appendix 3.

1. **In a cohort of patients with septic shock and high risk of mortality, our open-label use of esmolol after initial hemodynamic optimization resulted in maintenance of heart rate within the target range of 80/min to 94/min.[32]**

2. **Use of lung function to characterize severity is, currently, the best system available to clinicians, but it clearly falls well short of being ideal.[33]**

3. **The response to many drugs in common use varies greatly among patients.[34]**

4. **These agents seem to facilitate the use of shortened courses of combination interferon-free therapy, which are associated with high (>95%) sustained response rates and relatively few toxicities.[35]**

5. **Lactate levels have become a useful marker for tissue hypoperfusion and may also serve as an end point for resuscitation in patients with sepsis and septic shock.[36]**

6. Women with hypothyroidism should be counseled about the importance of achieving euthyroidism before conception because of the risk of decreased fertility and miscarriage.[37]

Conclusion

This chapter gave tips on preferring concrete language. Change an abstract subject into a concrete subject. Use nouns and verbs to carry the weight of meaning, instead of adjectives and adverbs. Write in the singular. Talk in terms of one doctor treating one patient.

In the next chapter, we talk about how to choose the right word so your reader can tell right away whether you are talking about something abstract or concrete.

Notes

1. *Wiktionary*, s.v. "Abstract," https://en.wiktionary.org/wiki/abstract (accessed December 2, 2014).
2. Gadalla S, et al. "Association between Donor Leukocyte Telomere Length and Survival After Unrelated Allogeneic Hematopoietic Cell Transplantation for Severe Aplastic Anemia," *JAMA* 313, no. 6 (2015): 600.
3. Mannino, "Global Burden of COPD," 766 (see chap. 1, n. 8).
4. Furie, "Do Pharmacogenetics Have a," 2345 (see chap. 2, n. 30).
5. Mallett, "Systematic Reviews of Diagnostic," under "Introduction" (see chap. 1, n. 18).
6. Yang, "Association of Dysglycemia and," 931 (see chap. 3, n. 18).
7. Kodner C, Wetherton A, "Diagnosis and Management of Physical Abuse in Children," *Am Fam Phys* 88, no. 10 (2013): 673.
8. Carney, "Thyroid Disease in Pregnancy," 273 (see chap. 3, n. 19).
9. Kawwass, "Trends and Outcomes for," 2427 (see chap. 4, n. 27).
10. Mannino, "Global Burden of COPD," 766 (see chap. 1, n. 8).
11. Furie, "Do Pharmacogenetics Have a," 2345 (see chap. 2, n. 30).
12. Jorgensen, "Effect of Screening and," under "Introduction" (see chap. 1, n. 10).
13. Sim J, et al. "Characteristics of Resistant Hypertension in a Large, Ethnically Diverse Hypertension Population of an Integrated Health System," *Mayo Clinic Proc* 88, no. 10 (2013): 1101.
14. Zolotor A, Carlough M, "Update on Prenatal Care," *Am Fam Phys* 79, no. 3 (2014): 199.
15. Strunk, *The Elements of Style*, 71 (see chap. 4, n. 2).
16. Liberman M, "Stop Hating on Adjectives and Adverbs," *Slate.com*, September 10, 2013, http://www.slate.com/blogs/lexicon_valley/2013/09/10/adjectives_and_adverbs_mark_twain_suggested_killing_them_but_counting_modifiers.html.
17. Alfandre, "What is Wrong with," 2393 (see chap. 1, n. 7).
18. Wang, "Age-Specific and Sex-Specific Mortality," 2072 (see chap. 1, n. 24).
19. Weinshilbourn, "Inheritance and Drug Response," 530 (see chap. 1, n. 17).
20. Mallett, "Systematic Reviews of Diagnostic," under "Introduction" (see chap. 1, n. 18).
21. Silber, "Willis Ekbom Disease Foundation," 977 (see chap. 3, n. 12).
22. Pelkowski, "Celiac Disease: Diagnosis and," 104 (see chap. 1, n. 21).
23. Bryan Garner, seminar in the early 1990s.
24. Smith D, *The Hundred and One Dalmatians*, (London: Heinemann, 1956).
25. *Wikipedia*, s.v. "Singular They," https://en.wikipedia.org/wiki/Singular_they (accessed February 23, 2016).

26. Chen, "Low-Dose Dopamine or," 2534 (see chap. 4, n. 15).
27. Mannino, "Global Burden of COPD," 766 (see chap. 1, n. 8).
28. Caraco, "Genes and the Response," 2867 (see chap. 2, n. 43).
29. Jorgensen, "Effect of Screening and," under "Intervention" (see chap. 1, n. 10).
30. Yang, "Association of Dysglycemia and," 931 (see chap. 3, n. 18).
31. Yew, "Diagnostic Approach to Patients," 106 (see chap. 4, Table 4-2).
32. Morelli, "Effect of Heart Rate," 1688 (see chap. 1, Table 1-1).
33. Mannino, "Global Burden of COPD," 766 (see chap. 1, n. 8).
34. Caraco, "Genes and the Response," 2867 (see chap. 2, n. 43).
35. Feeney, "Antiviral Treatment of Hepatitis," under "Abstract" (see chap. 3, n. 5).
36. Andersen L, et al. "Etiology and Therapeutic Approach to Elevated Lactate Levels," *Mayo Clinic Proc* 88, no. 10 (2013): 1129.
37. Carney, "Thyroid Disease in Pregnancy," 273 (see chap. 3, n. 19).

CHAPTER 6

Observe the 1066 principle

The truth is, many journal editors and senior scientists believe that unclear scientific writing is a serious problem.—Anne Greene, *Writing Science in Plain English*[1]

Introduction

In English, we tend to use short words to talk about the real world and longer words, more sparingly, to talk about abstract ideas. We call this tendency *the 1066 principle*. It applies to all kinds of writing, including medical writing. Observing the 1066 principle can help an author write more vividly.

How did English get to be this way? In 1066, William, Duke of Normandy, invaded England together with thousands of French-speaking knights, soldiers, clerks and clergy. These Norman invaders only partly replaced the existing English aristocracy. As a result, over the next few centuries, people living in England used Anglo-Saxon (Old English) and Norman French side by side. Eventually, French died out as a spoken language in England, while Anglo-Saxon took on many French words. Modern English emerged in the late 1400's as the London dialect became standard and the printing press came to England.[2]

The great sorting out

As the Normans brought French words into everyday use in England, there was often an Anglo-Saxon word with the same meaning. In some cases, English kept one word and dropped the other. In other cases, English kept both words, but gave each a slightly different meaning.[3] We generalize about this great sorting out in Table 6-1.

Let's look at examples of the 1066 principle at work in modern English. See Table 6-2. For each pair of words with a similar meaning, we use the short word to talk about the real world and the longer word to talk figuratively or about a more abstract idea.

Table 6-1. **Anglo-Saxon & Norman French words**

Anglo-Saxon	Norman French
basic meaning	specialized meaning
shorter words	longer words
literal	figurative
real-world	abstract
vivid	logical

Table 6-2. **Real world vs. abstract**

General idea	Real world	Abstract
Put on top	Heinz and Hilda *put* the tablecloth *on* the table.	The GM Canada logo *superimposes* a maple leaf over the GM logo.
Drink	John went to the pub to *drink* beer.	Sofia goes to the library to *imbibe* knowledge.
What's left?	Nick ate half the pizza and put *the rest* in the refrigerator.	80 divided by 7 equals 11 with a *remainder of* 3.
Subtract	If I *have* four apples and I *eat* one, how many do I *have left*?	How much is four *minus* one? Four *minus* one *equals* three.
Watering	Betsy *watered* her flowers.	Manuel *irrigated* the fields.

WATER VS. IRRIGATE

Looking at the last example in Table 6-2, you might ask, isn't irrigating a field a real-world activity? It does involve putting real water on real plants. But to irrigate a field, whether in ancient Egypt or modern China, an engineer must do several things: determine the water needs for the crop; find a stable water source; plan and build a system of canals, pipes, and pumps to move the water from the source to the fields, etc. If we consider these steps, we see irrigating a field is not just a real-world activity. It involves complex activities guided by abstract planning and analysis.

THE 1066 PRINCIPLE APPLIES TO MATH

Medical writing often deals with math or statistics. We tend to state a story problem in real-world terms. For example, "If I *have* two mice in the cage, and I *buy* two more mice, then how many mice do I *have*?" When we talk about math in the abstract, we use longer French or Latin-origin words (e.g., *plus, minus,*

Table 6-3. **Three ways to state a math problem**

Story problem in real-world terms	Abstract in words	Abstract in symbols
A surgical team operates on Bob. If they *start with* 12 sponges before the surgery, but *count* only 11 after the surgery, how many sponges did they *leave inside* Bob?	12 *minus* 11 *equals* ____.	12 – 11 = ____
If the field hospital has 12 tents to house 103 Ebola patients, how many patients must share each tent?	103 *divided* by 12 *equals* ____.	103 ÷ 12 = ____

equals, divide, remainder, quotient, mode, median, standard deviation, frequency, distribution).

We can often state a math problem three ways: as a real-world story problem, as an abstract math problem in words, or as an abstract math equation in symbols. Stating the problem in symbols makes it less vivid, but easier to solve. See Table 6-3.

A. Prefer the short word to describe the real world

We can observe the 1066 principle at work in medical writing. In Table 5-1, in Chapter 5, we looked at examples of medical terms that deal with the real world or the world of abstract ideas. The words in the *Real world* column tend to be short—mostly one or two syllables.[4] There are also some longer terms, but they tend to be names or essential scientific terms: *artery, arteriole, biopsy, injection, ovary, stethoscope, testicle* and *thermometer.*

The words in the *World of abstract ideas* column tend to be longer—three or more syllables.[5] Most are not essential scientific terms, since we can often find a way to say something similar in shorter, more concrete sounding words (e.g., *mortality/ death rate, circulation/ blood flow, surgical procedure/ operation, arrhythmia/ abnormal rhythm*).

Exercise 6.A. Prefer the short word to describe the real world
For each sentence:

1. Read it out loud and underline any <u>long word</u>. Double underline any word you consider an essential scientific term.
2. Does the sentence describe the real world? If so, revise to use short words to replace any long word other than an essential scientific term. Make any other changes you can think of to improve reading ease.

Compare your answers to the Exercise Key in Appendix 3.

> 1. **Herpes Zoster (HV), caused by the reactivation of latent varicella-zoster virus (VZV) manifests as an acute, painful vesicular rash and is often accompanied by chronic pain or postherpetic neuralgia.**[6]
>
> 2. **Fifth, the airflow limitation or obstruction that happens in COPD is caused by a mixture of small airway disease, parenchymal destruction (emphysema), and, in many cases, increased airways responsiveness (asthma).**[7]
>
> 3. **Maintenance of nocturnal euglycemia is extremely important and is challenging, since most cases of severe hypoglycemia occur at night.**[8]
>
> 4. **Similarly, patients with diabetes had a lower risk of arterial thrombosis than those without diabetes.**[9]
>
> 5. **Immune responses are orchestrated by a complex, continually evolving cooperative network of mobile cells and their products.**[10]
>
> 6. **The initial workup for urticaria and angioedema is a history and physical examination to determine a possible etiology.**[11]

B. Prefer 's to show real-world possession or connection

In English, we have a few different ways to show possession or connection. We tend to use the 's ending to show real-world possession or connection. We tend to use *of* to show abstract possession or connection. We also sometimes use other word endings, or no word ending at all. But open any medical journal today and you rarely find an 's. This is a symptom of *medicus incomprehensibilis*, which results from overusing abstract language.

Let's look at some examples of real-world and abstract possession or connection. See Table 6-4.

WHEN IS IT BETTER TO USE *OF*?

We recommend using *of* sparingly. For example, when you're talking about something abstract and it doesn't sound right to use 's, because it sounds too literal.

Sir Arthur Conan Doyle was an ophthalmologist who published his first medical article, *Gelsemium as a Poison* in the *British Medical Journal* in 1879.[12] Sir Arthur is better known for creating the most famous fictional characters of all time, Sherlock Holmes and Dr. Watson.

Sir Arthur's most famous Sherlock Holmes novel is called, *The Hound of the Baskervilles*. Why didn't he call the novel, *The Baskervilles' Hound*, using s' to show real-world possession or connection? Because one of the book's mysteries is

Table 6-4. **Real-world vs. abstract possession or connection**

Example	Abstract or real-world?
The doctor's white coat hangs on the door.	Real world
The patient's blood pressure was high.	Real world
The nurse ignored the patient's complaint *of* pain.	This implies the patient's complaint is real, but their pain might not be.
The nurse ignored the patient's pain complaint.	This implies the patient's complaint and pain are real.
The objectives *of* the current study were to identify distinct sets of functional trajectories in the year immediately before and after a serious fall injury, to evaluate the relationship between the prefall and postfall trajectories, and to determine whether these results differed based on the type *of* injury, namely hip fracture vs. other serious fall injuries.[i]	An *objective* is an abstract idea. It is appropriate to say, the *objectives of the study*, but we could also say, *the current study's objectives*. A *type of injury* is an abstract idea. It would sound awkward to say, *the injury's type*.

[i]Gill T, et al. "The Course of Disability Before and After a Serious Fall Injury," *JAMA Intern Med* 173, no. 19 (2013): 1781.

whether or not the hound really exists. The title, *The Hound of the Baskervilles,* leaves open the possibility the hound might just be a legend.

As a medical writer, you rarely want to sound vague or tantalize your reader with a mystery. Instead, you want to present your ideas clearly and directly. Favoring *'s* to show real-world possession or connection is one useful tool.

Exercise 6.B. Prefer 's to show real-world possession or connection
For each sentence:

1. Read it out loud and underline each word or word ending that shows <u>possession</u> or <u>connection</u>. Tell whether that possession or connection relates to the real world or the world of abstract ideas.
2. Revise to drop any unnecessary word ending. Show real-world possession using *'s*. Make any other changes you can think of to improve reading ease.

Compare your answers to the Exercise Key in Appendix 3.

1. Within each of these 2 cohorts, we compared the effectiveness of each intervention with a control (sleep hygiene informational video).[13]

2. **In this report and the accompanying appendix, we present the data, methods and key findings of the Global Burden of Disease Study 2010 on levels, trends, and age patterns of mortality worldwide.**[14]

3. **Importantly, these trials all examine the initiation of therapy with vitamin K antagonists and use as a primary end point the percentage of time that a patient is within the therapeutic range during the initial phase of treatment.**[15]

4. **Systematic reviews of diagnostic studies involve additional challenges to those of therapeutic studies.**[16]

5. **Randomized clinical trials are essential to evaluate therapies that reduce rather than eliminate a complication of a disease.**[17]

6. **The U.S. Preventive Services Task Force recommends routine HIV screening, known as opt-out screening, regardless of patient or physician perception of risk for all persons 15 to 65 years of age, unless a patient refuses.**[18]

C. Use terms consistently; avoid elegant variation

For medical writing, precise meaning and clear understanding are vital. You may have learned in school to vary terms to make your writing more interesting. This is called, *elegant variation.*[19] Elegant variation is used when reading ease is not a concern and there is no possibility of confusion. For example, if you write a report about Thomas Edison, you might refer to him as *the Wizard of Menlo Park,* so you don't keep saying, *Edison did this,* and *Edison did that.*

As with other types of technical writing, there is little place for elegant variation in medical writing. You will potentially confuse your reader if you use different terms for the same concept. For example, if you use the term *senior citizens* to refer to a group, continue to use this term throughout your article. Don't substitute another term, such as *the elderly* or *the aged.* Using a different term may cause the reader to wonder if you are referring to the same group.

Don't feel you need to use synonyms to make your writing more interesting. While using different words may make writing more interesting, it may decrease clarity.[20]

Elegant variation often violates the 1066 principle by pairing a concrete-sounding word with an abstract-sounding word, or by using words with different levels of abstraction. Either situation can confuse a reader.

Exercise 6.C. Use terms consistently; avoid elegant variation
For each sentence:

1. Read it out loud and underline any place in the text that talks about a similar idea using different terms.
2. Revise to use consistent terms. Make any other changes you can think of to improve reading ease.

Compare your answers to the Exercise Key in Appendix 3.

1. Portenoy states the problem is a lack of studies, not positive results. Even though there is minimal literature on long-term efficacy of opioids for chronic noncancer pain, the few studies that have been published have failed to find good evidence for efficacy.[21]

2. Estimates from WHO's Global Burden of Disease and Risk Factors project show that in 2001, COPD was the fifth leading cause of death in high-income countries, accounting for 3.8% of total deaths, and it was the sixth leading cause of death in nations of low and middle income, accounting for 4.9% of total deaths.[22]

3. Many legislatures and regulatory boards have adopted model pain statutes that encourage compliance with established standards for prescribing of pharmacologic agents for pain and other symptoms and that protect physicians who observe these guidelines from regulatory intrusion and possible prosecution.[23]

4. With the emergence of new direct acting antivirals, the treatment paradigm for hepatitis C virus (HCV) infection is currently undergoing its greatest change since the discovery of the virus 25 years ago. New data are routinely released for different combinations of these new agents, each reporting exceptionally high sustained response rates for an infection that was once notoriously difficult to treat. It is therefore difficult (even for those practicing in the field) to keep abreast of present treatment options, or what is likely to be available in the next 12–18 months. Because newer antivirals have recently been licensed in the United States and Europe, and the results of several promising large phase III studies have been recently published, now is an opportune time to review the current treatment landscape for HCV, and to anticipate how that landscape might look in coming years.[24]

5. Men taking zolpidem are at an increased risk of major injury. Compared with the corresponding comparison cohort, the male zolpidem user cohort had a higher risk of major injury.[25]

6. Celiac disease occurs in persons of European ancestry and in those of Middle Eastern, Indian, South American, and North African descent. It is rare in persons of Asian descent.[26]

D. Avoid using a long, Latin word to describe the real world

Traditional medical writing sometimes ignores the 1066 principle by (1) using a long word that sounds abstract to talk about the real world, or (2) using a short word that sounds concrete to talk about something abstract. Either one can confuse a reader by giving a *false signal* of *abstract* or *real world*.

FALSE-SIGNAL WORDS

Let's consider some examples of *false-signal words*. Traditional medical writing uses the terms *mediate, modulate* and *regulate* to describe real-world, natural processes. But, in common usage, these same words are mostly used to describe a complex activity guided by human thought and analysis. (For example, "the Securities and Exchange Commission *regulates* the stock market.")

Consider the example in Table 6-5, which uses the terms *mediated* and *modulated*. The false-signal words *mediate* and *modulate* help make this sentence seem "abstract" or "theoretical." (But nothing is more real-world than the way Fentanyl acts in a patient's body.)

The mixed message about whether Fentanyl *mediates* or *modulates* the patient's response to pain adds to the problem. By revising to eliminate the false-signal words *mediate* and *modulate,* we can give this sentence a more "real-world" feel. This makes the discussion clearer and easier to follow.

Social psychologists also use the terms *mediator* and *moderator* to describe real-world factors that affect a person's behavior. A 1986 journal article notes that psychology researchers tend to get these terms mixed up. It then goes on for eight pages explaining their proper use.[27]

Table 6-6 lists terms to describe when a person can perceive a stimulus. These long words look abstract, but each talks about a real-world natural process. As Table 6-6 shows, we can easily paraphrase in plain English.

Often, you can replace a word that sounds abstract with other words that sound more concrete. If you need ideas on how to do this, try looking up forms of *mediate, modulate* and *regulate* in *Stedman's Medical Dictionary.*[28]

Table 6-5. **Revising to minimize false signal words**

Original	*Revised*
Fentanyl-<u>mediated</u> or <u>modulated</u> responses involve action at the μ-opioid receptor as an agonist at the dorsal horn inhibiting ascending pain pathways in the rostral ventral medulla, increasing pain threshold, and producing both analgesic and sedative effects.[i] (WSEG = 36/36.0/0.0/23.6)	Fentanyl acts on the μ-opioid receptor as an agonist at the dorsal horn. This action inhibits ascending pain pathways in the rostral ventral medulla. The result is to increase the patient's pain threshold, reduce their pain, and calm them. (WSEG = 39/13.0 /56.9/8.5)

[i]Ruan X, Chiravuri S, Kaye A, "Toxicological Testing when Evaluating Cases of Suspected of Acute Fentanyl Toxicity," *Forensic Sci Med Pathol* (July 7, 2016).

Table 6-6. **Sense of perception**

Long Latin terms	Plain English (sense of____)
ophthalmoception	sight
audioception	hearing
gustaoception	taste
olfacoception or olfacception	smell
tactioception	touch
nociception	pain
equilibrioception	balance
thermoception	warmth
proprioception	one's own movement

SUMMARY

English tends to use long Latin words, sparingly, to talk about abstract ideas. Because of this, long words tend to signal *abstract*. Using a long word to talk about the real world tends to confuse by sending a false signal.

If you want to write clearly, try to avoid false signal words. This helps make your writing more vivid and easier for a reader to follow. It also helps break down the walls that hamper the free flow of ideas between fields.

Exercise 6.D. Avoid using a long, Latin word to describe the real world
For each sentence:

1. Read it out loud. Underline the words *mediate*, *modulate* or *regulate* whenever they appear in any form (e.g., *regulatory*).
2. Tell whether you think the sentence describes the real world or an abstract idea. If you think the sentence describes the real world, revise to use shorter or more concrete-sounding words. Make any other changes you can think of to improve reading ease.

Compare your answers to the Exercise Key in Appendix 3.

> **1. The risk of HZ is elevated by 1.5 to 2 times in patients with rheumatic and immune-mediated diseases such as rheumatoid arthritis (RA) and Crohn's disease.**[29]

Note: *HZ* stands for *Herpes Zoster*.

> **2. We hypothesise that rare ADRB2 variants modulate therapeutic responses to LABA therapy and contribute to rare, severe adverse events.**[30]

Note: *ADRB2* stands for the β_2 *adrenergic receptor gene.* *LABA* stands for *long acting β antagonist.*

> **3. Among the 54 patients, we identified 5 who could willfully modulate their brain activity (Figure 1).**[31]
>
> **4. Transparency of the regulatory system is also required to overcome several dysfunctions in the drug industry's behaviour.**[32]
>
> **5. Some experimental support exists for the concept that the ability to discriminate between "self" and "nonself" involves learning to respond aggressively when there are signals that suggest the presence of invasive pathogens and having effective regulatory mechanisms for suppressing inflammatory responses when such signals are absent.**[33]
>
> **6. Urticaria and angioedema are thought to have similar underlying pathophysiological mechanisms, with histamine and other mediators being released from mast cells and basophils.**[34]

Conclusion

Remember the 1066 principle. If you want to make your writing easier to understand, talk about the real world using short words. Use long words, sparingly, to talk about abstract ideas. Use 's to show real-world possession or connection or to show abstract possession or connection if it sounds okay. Avoid the elegant variation.

Notes

1. Greene, *Writing Science in Plain,* 1 (see Preface, n. 7).
2. Baugh A, Cable T, *A History of the English Language,* 5th ed. (London: Prentice-Hall, 2002), 67–115.
3. Thus, e.g., in modern English, we use Anglo-Saxon-origin words, *cow, calf, pig* and *sheep,* to talk about the animal, and French-origin words, *beef, veal, pork,* and *mutton,* to talk about the food.
4. Some are Anglo-Saxon origin: heart, heartbeat, blood, flow, beat, pill, shot, dies, death, gut, lung, cough, egg, and womb. Some are short French or Latin-origin: vein, IV bolus, tumor, cancer, spinal cord, urine and sample.
5. Most are French or Latin origin; only a few are Anglo-Saxon.
6. Zhang J, et al. "Association between Vaccination for Herpes Zoster and Risk of Herpes Zoster Infection among Older Patients with Selected Immune-Mediated Diseases," *JAMA* 308, no. 1 (2012): 43.
7. Mannino, "Global Burden of COPD," 766 (see chap. 1, n. 8).
8. Phillip M, et al. "Nocturnal Glucose Control with an Artificial Pancreas at Diabetes Camp," *N Eng J Med* 368 (2013): 825.

9. Donzé J, et al. "Impact of Sepsis on Risk of Postoperative Arterial and Venous Thromboses: Large Prospective Cohort Study," *BMJ* 349 (2014), under "Subgroup Analysis for Arterial Thrombosis," http://www.bmj.com/content/349/bmj.g5334.
10. Carter, "B Cells in Health," under "Article Outline," (see Concept 1, n. 8).
11. Schaefer P, "Urticaria: Evaluation and Treatment," *Am Fam Phys* 83, no. 9 (2011), under "Evaluation," http://www.aafp.org/afp/2011/0501/p1078.html.
12. *Wikipedia*, s.v. "Arthur Conan Doyle," https://en.wikipedia.org/wiki/Arthur_Conan_Doyle (accessed June 15, 2015).
13. Kravitz, "Patient Engagement Programs for," 1819 (see chap. 4, Table 4–1).
14. Wang, "Age-specific and Sex-specific Mortality," 2072 (see chap. 1, n. 24).
15. Furie, "Do Pharmacogenetics Have a," 2346 (see chap. 2, n. 30).
16. Mallett, "Systematic Reviews of Diagnostic," under "Introduction" (see chap. 1, n. 18).
17. Sniderman A, et al. "The Necessity for Clinical Reasoning in the Era of Evidence-Based Medicine," *Mayo Clinic Proc* 88, no. 10 (2013): 1108.
18. Sherin K, et al. "What is New in HIV Infection?" *Am Fam Phys* 89, no. 4 (2014): 265.
19. Folwer H W, quoted in Garner B, *The Elements of Legal Style* (Oxford: Oxford University Press, 1991), 205–206.
20. Plain Language Action and Information Network, *Federal Plain Language Guidelines*, 45 (see chap. 4, n. 4).
21. Dowell D, Kunins H, Farley T, "Letters: In Reply," *JAMA* 310, no. 16 (2013): 1738.
22. Mannino, "Global Burden of COPD," 765 (see chap. 1, n. 8).
23. Quill, "The Big Chill: Inserting," 1 (see chap. 3, n. 16).
24. Feeney, "Antiviral Treatment of Hepatitis," under "Introduction" (see chap. 3, n. 5).
25. Lai, "Long-Term Use of Zolpidem," 593 (see chap. 4, n. 19).
26. Pelkowski, "Celiac Disease: Diagnosis and," 99 (see chap. 1, n. 21).
27. Baron R, Kenny D, "The Moderator-Mediator Variable Distinction in Social Psychological Research: Conceptual, Strategic, and Statistical Considerations," *Journal of Personality and Social Psychology* 51, no. 6 (1986), 1173.
28. *Stedman's Medical Dictionary*, s.v. "Mediate."
29. Zhang, "Association between Vaccination for," 43 (see chap. 6, n. 6).
30. Ortega V, et al. "Effect of Rare Variants in ADRB2 on Risk of Severe Exacerbations and Symptom Control During Long Acting β Agonist Treatment in a Multiethnic Asthma Population: A Genetic Study," *Lancet Resp Med* 2, no. 3 (2014), under "Background," http://www.thelancet.com/journals/lanres/articles/PIIS2213-2600(13)70289-3/fulltext.
31. Monti M, et al. "Willful Modulation of Brain Activity in Disorders of Consciousness," *N Eng J Med* 362 (2010), under "Results," http://www.nejm.org/doi/full/10.1056/NEJMoa0905370.
32. Garattini S, Bertele V, "Europe's Opportunity to Open Up Drug Regulation," *BMJ* 340 (2010), under "Transparency as a Means to Avoid Bias," http://www.bmj.com/content/340/bmj.c1578.
33. Carter, "B Cells in Health," under "The Immune System and B Cells Form and Function" (see Concept 1, n. 8).
34. Schaefer, "Urticaria: Evaluation and Treatment," under "Etiology" (see chap. 6, n. 11).

CHAPTER *7*

Statistical analysis of *WSEG* scores

Everything should be made as simple as possible, but not simpler.
—Albert Einstein

Introduction

At the start of this book, we identified symptoms of *medicus incomprehensibilis*. The tips in Chapters 1–6 addressed those symptoms related to low reading ease and needless abstraction. The exercises in these chapters used medical journal excerpts that showed at least one symptom. In the Exercise Key, we gave our revisions and before-and-after *WSEG* scores.

In this chapter, we give our analysis of these *WSEG* scores. The original excerpts had an average sentence length of 30.1 words, a 13.4 reading ease score, and an 18.6 grade level. Our revisions had an average sentence length of 14.1 words, a 57.9 reading ease score, and an 8.6 grade level. This analysis provides evidence you can treat *medicus incomprehensibilis* effectively by applying the tips in this book.

Figures 7-1 through 7-4 show the breakdown of *WSEG* scores. The top part of each figure shows the raw scores.[1] The bottom part shows the mean of all scores. For Figures 7-2 through 7-4, we also show the ranges around the mean where most scores fall. We show the range of plus or minus one standard deviation ($\mu \pm 1\sigma$), where 67% of scores fall. We also show the range of plus or minus two standard deviations ($\mu \pm 2\sigma$), where 95% of scores fall.

Analysis

TOTAL WORDS (*w*)

Figure 7-1 shows the distribution of total words. Total words for the originals is shown in black. Total words for our revisions is shown in stripe. Total words changed only slightly in our revisions.

The original excerpts had a mean of 34.2 words; our revisions had a mean of 34.8 words. But since we replaced long words with short ones where we could, our revisions tend to take up slightly less space on the page.

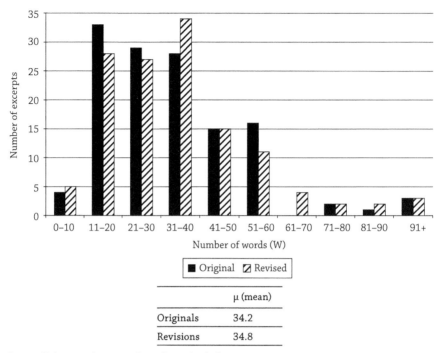

Figure 7-1 Distribution of total words *(W)*

SENTENCE LENGTH (S)

Figure 7-2 shows the distribution of sentence lengths for the originals and our revisions. The mean sentence length for the originals was 30.1 words. Sentence lengths in the originals were widely distributed. The range of plus or minus one standard deviation ran from 15.7 to 44.4 words per sentence. The range of plus or minus two standard deviations ran from 1.3 to 58.8 words per sentence.

The mean sentence length for our revisions was 14.1 words. Sentence lengths for our revisions were more narrowly distributed. The range of plus or minus one standard deviation ran from 10.8 to 17.4 words per sentence. The range of plus or minus two standard deviations ran from 7.6 to 20.7 words per sentence.

Overall, our revisions greatly reduced average sentence length. Even the high end of our 95% range (20.7 words per sentence) was lower than the mean of the originals (30.1 words per sentence).

READING EASE (E)

Figure 7-3 shows the distribution of reading ease scores for the originals and our revisions. This distribution includes negative reading ease scores.[2]

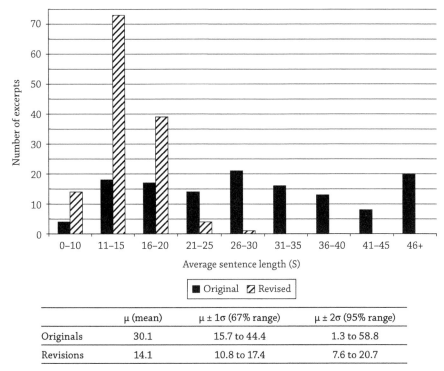

	μ (mean)	μ ± 1σ (67% range)	μ ± 2σ (95% range)
Originals	30.1	15.7 to 44.4	1.3 to 58.8
Revisions	14.1	10.8 to 17.4	7.6 to 20.7

Figure 7-2 Distribution of average sentence length *(S)*

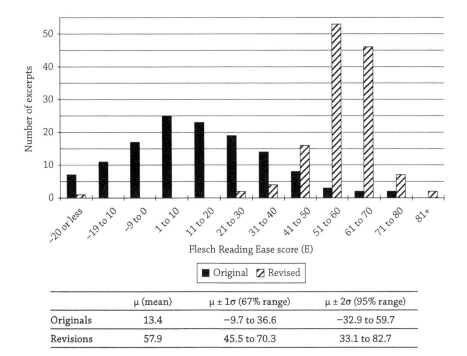

	μ (mean)	μ ± 1σ (67% range)	μ ± 2σ (95% range)
Originals	13.4	−9.7 to 36.6	−32.9 to 59.7
Revisions	57.9	45.5 to 70.3	33.1 to 82.7

Figure 7-3 Distribution of reading ease scores *(E)*

The mean reading ease score for the originals was 13.4. Reading ease scores for the originals were widely distributed. The range of plus or minus one standard deviation ran from a reading ease score of −9.7 to 36.6. The range of plus or minus two standard deviations ran from a reading ease score of −32.9 to 59.7.

The mean reading ease score for our revisions was 57.9. The reading ease scores for our revisions were more narrowly distributed. The range of plus or minus one standard deviation ran from a reading ease score of 45.5 to 70.3. The range of plus or minus two standard deviations ran from a reading ease score of 33.1 to 82.7. The low end of our 95% range (a 33.1 reading ease score) was much higher than the mean of the originals (13.4).

GRADE LEVEL (G)

Figure 7-4 shows the distribution of grade levels for the originals and our revisions. The mean grade level for the originals was 18.6. A non-native English speaker may have an 18th-grade level knowledge of science, but their knowledge of English may not be at the same level.

The grade levels for the originals were widely distributed. The range of plus or minus one standard deviation ran from a grade level of 12.9 to 24.3. The range of plus or minus two standard deviations ran from a grade level of 7.2 to 29.9.

The mean grade level for our revisions was 8.6. This grade level seems more appropriate for a typical non-native speaker (e.g., think of a doctor from Europe,

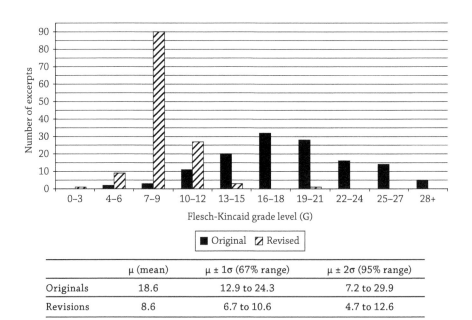

	μ (mean)	μ ± 1σ (67% range)	μ ± 2σ (95% range)
Originals	18.6	12.9 to 24.3	7.2 to 29.9
Revisions	8.6	6.7 to 10.6	4.7 to 12.6

Figure 7-4 Distribution of grade level scores (*G*)

Asia or Africa). Lowering the grade level by 10 school grades (8.6 vs. 18.6) should cut reading time and improve reading comprehension for all readers.

The grade levels for our revisions were more narrowly distributed. The range of plus or minus one standard deviation ran from a grade level of 6.7 to 10.6. The range of plus or minus two standard deviations ran from a grade level of 4.7 to 12.6. The high end of our 95% range (a grade level of 12.6) fell far below the mean of the originals (18.6).

Limitations

Of course, this analysis is not a formal study. Further research is needed (e.g., to quantify the savings in reading time). The excerpts do not represent a random sample of medical writing, nor do they represent medical writing as a whole.

Conclusion

We applied the tips in this book to the excerpts and greatly improved reading ease and grade level. Our revisions reflect what can reasonably be achieved when writing in plain English. Using the tips in this book can help medical authors eradicate *medicus incomprehensibilis.*

Exercise 7. Putting the tips on reading ease and vivid language into practice
Review the symptoms of *medicus incomprehensibilis* listed in Table I-1 in the Introduction. Read the excerpt from "The Frequency and Cost of Treatment Perceived to be Futile in Critical Care," out loud (Appendix 2, No. 2).

1. What symptoms of *medicus incomprehensibilis* do you see? Name at least five. Describe the symptoms or give examples.
2. Revise using the tips on reading ease and vivid language.

Compare your revision to the Exercise Key in Appendix 3.

Notes

1. Scores have been rounded to the nearest integer.
2. We computed negative reading ease scores using the Flesch Reading Ease and Flesch-Kincaid Grade Level formulas; see *Wikipedia,* s.v. "Flesch-Kincaid readability tests" https://en.wikipedia. org/wiki/Flesch%E2%80%93Kincaid_readability_tests (accessed March 28, 2016). The WSEG score gave us the data we needed to compute the reading ease score, except for total number of syllables. We found the total number of syllables, by using the grade level formula and solving for the number of syllables.

PRESENT LOGICAL REASONING CLEARLY

A problem well-put is half-solved.—John Dewey

The last part of this book deals with clear logical reasoning. Much of the logic of any medical research is set at the time the research project is approved. The outline for an article is set by the journal. Peer review checks the reasoning. The tips we give here relate to presenting information clearly to help minimize *medicus incomprehensibilis*.

The logic of a medical article is usually clear. Now and then, when it's not, you can still usually figure it out. But this may be your knowledge and experience as a reader compensating for an unclear article.

Example—The scrambled owner's manual

Imagine you've just presented your latest research at a medical conference in a tropical location. As you drive your rental car around the island, a tire goes flat. You decide to change it yourself, but you don't know where to find the spare or the jack. So you take out the owner's manual.

Suppose the owner's manual has good reading ease and uses vivid language, but the directions are in the wrong order. (For example, it tells you how to tighten a lug nut, before it tells you where to find the jack.) You puzzle over the directions. Under these circumstances, if you've changed a tire before, you can probably figure things out. But this is an instance of your knowledge and experience filling in for the owner's manual's poor organization.

This example shows two things. First, how a narrative is organized is a separate concept from reading ease or vivid language. Second, just because you can change a flat tire using a scrambled owner's manual, doesn't mean the manual is well-written; it ought to be written so anybody can change a flat tire. In the same way, just because an expert can get the information they need from an article doesn't mean it is well-written. It should be written for the widest reasonable audience.

Why save logic for last?

Why do we address logical reasoning last after reading ease and vivid language? For one thing, unclear logical reasoning makes the smallest contribution to *medicus incomprehensibilis*. The logic of a medical journal article is usually clear. The issues of logical flow we see now and then tend to be small. Perhaps a step of reasoning is missing or ideas are presented in a confusing order.

The second reason is, when you improve reading ease and make your language more vivid, it often helps reveal a problem with logical reasoning that may have been hidden.

The third reason is, it's more complicated. Logical reasoning is harder to discuss, since you need to look at bigger chunks of text—several sentences or paragraphs—not just one sentence. Because logic deals with both *substance* and *form*, you need to understand the science. You also need to understand what the author is trying to say.

Improving the flow of logical reasoning takes time and thought, but it's worth it. When you improve logic, you improve both style and content.

In the next three chapters, we give tips on presenting logical reasoning clearly.

8. Organize your narrative in a way that's helpful for your reader
9. Choose a clear narrative pathway
10. Forge a strong chain of logical reasoning

Overview of Concept 3 exercises

Since analyzing logic involves looking at bigger chunks of text, Concept 3 uses fewer exercises, and each exercise takes more thought. In Chapter 8, we look at paragraphs and ask you to consider how you might present the information in a way that is more helpful to the reader.

In Chapters 9 and 10, we look at an excerpt from *Mathematical Modeling of Kidney Transport*. We ask you to consider how you might adapt it reach a wider audience.

CHAPTER 8

Organize your narrative in a way that's helpful for your reader

Good paragraphs have unity. They have topic sentences that announce the idea to be developed in the paragraph, and then they stick to that idea. And headings can powerfully reinforce the unity of your paragraphs.—Bryan Garner[1]

A good narrative organizes information in a way that helps the reader. When a narrative fails to organize information well, it adds to *medicus incomprehensibilis*.

One failure we occasionally see is the overly long paragraph. Another is that a narrative presents two-dimensional data as one-dimensional standard prose. Either one of these writing habits places an unnecessary burden on the reader to analyze and interpret the information. This chapter covers simple strategies for treating these problems.

A. Introduce and develop one idea in each paragraph

A paragraph should start with a sentence that suggests the topic or helps with transition from the previous paragraph. Or else, it may tell about the new paragraph's function as part of the whole. If you start a paragraph with a good heading or topic sentence, it can help your reader quickly grasp that idea.[2]

Dividing a narrative into good paragraphs helps a reader see the progression of ideas. If a single paragraph goes on too long, it may shift the burden of seeing the progression of ideas over to the reader. The reader can no longer simply read the paragraph; instead, they have to study it.

A good paragraph heading or topic sentence is the reader's friend. If they ever want to look back to find something, they can do so quickly by looking at the headings or topic sentences.

How long should a paragraph be? Some authors advise that a writer should strive for an average paragraph of no more than 150 words, with a mixture of short and long paragraphs.[3]

Exercise 8.A. Introduce and develop one idea in each paragraph
For each excerpt:

1. Read it out loud. Do you understand it just by *reading* it, or do you need to *study* it?
2. Does it cover one idea or multiple ideas?
3. Without re-writing the text, split up the long paragraph into shorter paragraphs no more than 150 words each, covering just one idea or topic. Write a heading or topic sentence for each new paragraph.
4. In your view, do shorter paragraphs with headings or topic sentences make this excerpt easier to read? Why or why not?

Compare your answers with the Exercise Key in Appendix 3.

1. In a majority of cases, metabolism that is mediated by cytochrome P-450 represents a deactivation pathway. For some drugs, however, oxidation leads to conversion of a prodrug into an active compound. A prime example is codeine (metabolized by CYP2D6); other examples include clopidogrel (metabolized by CYP3A4), cyclophosphamide (metabolized by CYP2B6) and tamoxifen (metabolized by CYP2D6). The major pathway of codeine consists of glucuronidation and *N*-demethylation, whereas the CYP2D6-mediated *O*-demethylation to produce morphine is a minor reaction. Nevertheless, the latter is a crucial step in bioactivation, since the affinity of codeine for the μ-opioid receptor is only 1/200 to 1/3000 that of morphine. Previous studies have shown that the effects of codeine—analgesic, respiratory, psychomotor, and miotic—are markedly attenuated in people with poor metabolism of CYP2D6. On the other hand, people with ultrarapid metabolism, such as the patient described by Gasche et al. in this issue of the *Journal*, produce greater amounts of morphine from codeine and therefore may experience exaggerated pharmacologic effects in response to regular doses of codeine. Similar effects, albeit less dramatic, have been described in patients with ultrarapid metabolism of CYP2D6 in response to routine doses of hydrocodone or oxycodone, which are other opioids requiring CYP2D6 mediated activation. These reports clearly illustrate the effect of CYP2D6 genetic polymorphisms on the action of codeine, ranging from virtually no effect in patients with poor metabolism to severe toxic effects in those with ultrarapid metabolism. To put these observations into perspective, these extremes of response might be relevant for some 10 to 20 percent of whites who have phenotypes associated with either poor metabolism or ultrarapid metabolism.[4] *(WSEG = 269/29.8/10.9/18.4)*

2. The [pulmonary artery catheter] PAC, today still considered the clinical gold standard for CO estimation, gives three fundamental bits

of hemodynamic information: CO, pulmonary and cardiac filling pressures and mixed SvO_2. The PAC is considered the clinical gold standard or reference method for CO estimation and every new tool built for CO estimation has to be compared with PAC in validation studies. The technique is based on the injection of an ice-cold solution into the right atrium (proximal port—prox injectate—blue lumen). The change in blood temperature is measured in the pulmonary artery by a thermistor placed proximally to the tip of the catheter. The thermodilution curve is used for CO estimation by means of the Steward-Hamilton formulation. The measurement is repeated at least three to five times (in order to compensate for variations induced by the respiratory cycle) and the average value is then calculated. An "inverted" thermodilution curve can be obtained by worming [sic] the blood with a thermal filament (Vigilance™, Edwards Lifesciences, Irvine, CA, USA) or a thermal coil (OptiQ™, ICU Medical, San Clemente, CA, USA). This system allows for a semi-continuous CO measurement by displaying average CO values for the previous 10 min and limiting, for this reason, the effects of arrhythmias and other compounding factors. Although the CO value is frequently up-dated, this type of monitoring is not continuous (beat-by-beat) and is therefore less accurate and rapid in detecting hemodynamic instability. Major limiting factors for CO estimation with any type of thermodilution is the occurrence of tricuspid regurgitation and intracardiac shunts. In fact, prolonged indicator transit times or indicator recycling may lead to errors in CO estimation. SvO_2 suggests whether or not cardiac output is adequate in a patient since it provides a useful indication about the adequacy of tissue oxygenation in specific conditions of metabolic activity. When SvO_2 decreases below normal values (70–75%) in the presence of normal arterial oxygen saturation and without anemia, it means that CO is inadequate and measures aimed at increasing DO_2 should be promptly implemented. SvO_2 can be measured either continuously (fiberoptic fibers) or intermittently by withdrawing a mixed venous blood sample from the distal lumen of the PAC. The PAC measures: the pulmonary artery pressure which represents right ventricular afterload; right atrial pressure (RAP/CVP, PAOP) have been demonstrated to be less reliable than dynamic indicators of fluid responsiveness (pulse pressure variations PPV, systolic pressure variation SPV and stroke volume variation SVV). Nonetheless, when static parameters are particularly low, they can be considered to be as reliable as dynamic ones. Over recent years, the use of PAC has decreased significantly for two main reasons: firstly, several randomized and non-randomized studies have not demonstrated an improvement in patient outcomes when therapies were guided by PAC and secondly nowadays the PAC is the most invasive tool for hemodynamic monitoring currently used in ICUs or ORs. In 1996, Connors and co-workers published in *JAMA* a prospective cohort study in which the authors used case-matching multivariable regression modeling techniques and a propensity score. The results showed that pulmonary artery catheterization in critically ill patients was associated with an increased risk of death (odds ratio 1.24; 95% confidence interval 1.03–1.49) as well as a prolonged length of stay and increased resource utilization. After this shocking paper, a litany of randomized trials aimed at confirming these results was performed in ICUs. The net results of this great amount of data corresponded to an increased suspicion that PAC-guided treatment may not be superior to non-PAC-guided treatment and a marked decrease in PAC use worldwide has become clear during the last 10–15 years. In the USA, Wiener et al. reported a 65% decrease in PAC use between 1993 and 2004 and in Canada, Koo et al. reported a more than 50% decrease between 2002 and 2006. A great number of papers has been published by opinion leaders and general considerations about the use of PAC and its benefits. The doubts regarding its usefulness can be listed as follows.[5] *(WSEG = 667/27.7/18.5/17.0)*

B. Present two-dimensional data in a table, chart or graph

In any language, prose is one-dimensional. We write a string of words arranged in a line according to the order in which we speak them. English writes from left to right. Other languages write from right to left or top to bottom.

Unlike standard prose, some data is inherently two-dimensional. We can often understand a collection of data better if it's presented in a table, chart or graph. This often reduces the number of words, improves reading ease, and makes the data easier to grasp. (For example, when data is presented in a table, we sometimes choose to scan data down the columns, rather than across the rows.)

Let's consider an example:

Vasectomy reversal techniques involve reanastomosis of the testicular and prostatic vasal ends (vasovasostomy) or connecting the vas to the epididymis (vasoepididymostomy). Vasovasostomy patency rates have been reported between 75% and 86%; pregnancy rates range from 45% to 70%. Vasoepididymostomy, a technique used in the presence of epididymal obstruction, has patency rates between 31% and 92%, and pregnancy rates between 10% and 50%. Repeat attempts at microsurgical vasectomy reversal appear less successful than first attempts with patency rates between 75% and 79%, and pregnancy rates between 32% and 43%.[6] *(WSEG= 88/22.0/7.2/16.6)*

This subject, vasectomy reversal and pregnancy, has a high level of human interest, but the narrative sounds dull and reading ease is low. Why? It's partly due to long sentences and essential medical terms. It's also partly due to the fact that the data is presented in one-dimensional prose, which makes the reader have to work harder to understand. The data becomes easier to grasp if we organize it into a table. For example, we might summarize the same data as follows:

> Vasectomy reversal techniques involve re-attaching the testicle and prostate ends of the vas (*vasovasostomy*) or connecting the vas to the epididymis (*vasoepididymostomy*). Table 8-1 gives data on the reported outcomes for operations that use the different reversal techniques.

Table 8-1. **Outcomes for vasectomy reversal**

Procedure name	Procedure/indication	Success rate (%)	
		Vas freely open	*Pregnancy*
Vasovasotomy	Reconnect vas (prostate and testicle ends)	75–86	45–70
Vasoepididymostomy	Connect vas to epididymis, used when epididymis is blocked	31–92	10–50
Repeat attempts	Previous attempt to reconnect vas failed	75–79	32–43

The table helps the reader see three different types of information at a glance: (1) the procedures, (2) the possible success outcomes, and (3) the data that quantify the success rate.

Of course, creating a table requires the author to do more work. A table takes up more space on the page. But if you consider the value of the time saved for hundreds or thousands of readers, all busy professionals, the extra time and paper are certainly worth it.

For a good short discussion of creating effective tables, charts and graphs, we recommend, *The AMA Manual of Style,*[7] or *The Craft of Research* by Booth, Colomb and Williams.[8] For a more extensive discussion, consider the works of Edward Tufte.

SUMMARY

Presenting two-dimensional data in one-dimensional form often adds to *medicus incomprehensibilis.* Presenting data in two-dimensional form, as a table, chart or graph, can help treat the problem.

Exercise 8.B.   Present two-dimensional data in a table, chart or graph
For each sentence below:

1. Read it out loud. Underline any <u>data</u> you think might be clearer if presented in two-dimensional form.
2. Create a table or chart to present the data in two-dimensional form. Revise the remaining text to improve reading ease.

Compare your answers to the Exercise Key in Appendix 3.

> **1. All 525 study participants, who were randomized to receive vareni-cline or placebo, had been diagnosed with major depressive disorder and were being treated with antidepressant drugs at a stable dose or had been successfully treated for depression within the past 2 years. At 9 to 12 weeks, 35.9% of those who received varenicline quit vs. 15.6% taking placebo; at 40 weeks, 20.3% of the varenicline group had quit compared with 10.4% of the placebo group. Depression and anxiety did not increase in either group, but the researchers cautioned that their findings may not apply to smokers whose depression isn't successfully treated.[9]**

> **2. What about health in Scotland? According to the UK's national statistical office, healthy life expectancy was 59·8 years for men and 64·1 years for women in Scotland during 2008–10, 4·6 years and 2·3 years fewer than for men and women in England, respectively. According to the British Heart Foundation, 35% of Scottish men and 30% of women have high blood pressure; alcohol use is one noticeable contributor to ill health in Scotland, with up to 50% of men and 30% of women exceeding guidelines for drinking.[10]**

Conclusion

A good narrative organizes information in a way that helps the reader. In this chapter, we talked about two simple ways to organize information. Make sure a paragraph is not overly long and deals with just one subject. Use a heading or topic sentence to help preview the content for the reader. Organize two-dimensional data using a table, chart or graph. This allows the reader to grasp at a glance how each idea relates to the others.

In the next chapter, we look at *narrative pathway*.

Notes

1. Garner B, *Securities Disclosure in Plain English* (Chicago: CCH Incorporated, 1999), 64.
2. Strunk, *The Elements of Style*, 15–17 (see chap. 4, n. 2).
3. Garner, *Securities Disclosure in Plain*, 61–73.
4. Caraco, "Genes and the Response," 2868 (see chap. 2, n. 43).
5. Ramagnoli S, "Circulatory Failure: Exploring Macro- and Micro-Circulation," *Trends in Anaesthesia and Critical Care* 3 (2013), under "The Pulmonary Artery Catheter [PAC]," http://www.trendsanaesthesiacriticalcare.com/article/S2210-8440(13)00020-8/fulltext.
6. Rayala, "Common Questions about Vasectomy," 760 (see chap. 2, n. 7).
7. Iverson C, et al. ed. *AMA Manual of Style*, 10th ed. Oxford: Oxford University Press, 2007.
8. Booth W, Colomb G, Williams J, *The Craft of Research*, 3rd ed. (Chicago: University of Chicago Press, 2008); see chap. 15 on "Communicating Evidence Visually."
9. Slomski A, "Clinical Trials Update: Depression Remains Stable in Smokers Taking Varenicline to Quit," *JAMA* 310, no. 16 (2013): 1165.
10. "Scotland: Towards a Healthy and Interdependent Future," *Lancet* 384, no. 9947 (2014), http://www.thelancet.com/journals/;ancet/article/PIIS0140-6736(14)61614-7/fulltext.

CHAPTER 9

Choose a clear narrative pathway

If he would inform, he must advance regularly from Things known to things unknown, distinctly without Confusion, and the lower he begins the better. It is a common Fault in Writers, to allow their Reader too much knowledge: they begin with that which should be in the Middle, and skipping backwards and forwards, 'tis impossible for anyone but he who is perfect in the Subject before, to understand their Work, and such an one has no Occasion to read it.—Benjamin Franklin[1]

Why does an expert in their field talk over everybody's head? Why can't they talk about their subject in a simple way? Is it just because their ideas are too advanced or complex? Perhaps. But sometimes when an author understands their subject well, they become blind to what other people do or don't understand. They overestimate the reader's knowledge. They misjudge the widest reasonable audience, defining it too narrowly, composed of people just like themselves. As a result, they may do several things that confuse the reader.

1. They fail to start by talking about "things known."
2. They fail to start by anchoring their discussion in the real world.
3. They fail to follow a clear narrative pathway.
4. They make an abrupt transition between concrete and abstract or vice versa.

Narrative pathway is the direction of a narrative, or a conceptual program for organizing a narrative. Centuries ago, Benjamin Franklin saw that some people who wrote about science had a problem organizing their ideas. We see the same thing today. In this chapter, we give tips to avoid common problems and help you create a clear narrative pathway.

A. Start with things known

A good narrative often starts by stating things commonly known. Before talking about new discoveries developed through research, a medical article starts by talking about prior research and current knowledge and practice. For example, the article, "Effect of Aspirin and Antiplatelet Drugs on the Outcome of the Fecal Immunochemical Test," begins by reviewing facts about colorectal cancer and common screening techniques.

> Colorectal cancer (CRC) is the third most common cancer worldwide and the second leading cause of cancer-related deaths. Evidence from several studies has indicated that CRC screening is effective and cost-effective in average-risk populations. Recommended CRC screening strategies fall in 2 broad categories: stool tests that primarily detect cancer, which include detection of occult blood or exfoliated DNA, and structural tests, such as flexible signoidoscopy, colonoscopy, and computed tomographic colonography, which are effective in detecting both cancer and premalignant lesions.[2]

Exercise 9.A.   Start with things known
Review the excerpt *Mathematical Modeling of Kidney Transport* in Appendix 2.

> Do you think it starts by talking about concepts familiar to the widest reasonable audience? Why or why not?

Compare your answer to the Exercise Key in Appendix 3.

B. Start by anchoring your discussion in the real world

Starting with things known often involves starting in the real word. In Chapter 5, we saw how a sentence that uses a concrete subject is more vivid and easier to understand. The same concept applies to logical reasoning. People usually find the real world easier to grasp than an abstract idea. Science writing often proceeds from talking about research data (*real-world facts*) to analyzing them and drawing conclusions (*abstract analysis*).

Medical articles start with an abstract that summarizes the research. A reader often reads the abstract to decide whether to read the article. Therefore, it helps if the abstract is stated in real-world terms.

Consider two excerpts from the abstract of a recommendation statement by the US Preventative Services Task Force (Table 9–1). The statement covers the issue of whether a doctor should screen vision for an older patient. The original statement is not hard to understand, but it sounds formal and abstract. In particular, the term "visual acuity" (literally, sharpness or clearness of seeing) seems an abstract way to describe how well a patient sees things in the real world.

Table 9-1. **Start by anchoring the discussion in the real world**

Original[i]	*Revised*
DESCRIPTION Update of the US Preventive Services Task Force (USPSTF) recommendation on screening for impaired visual acuity in older adults. (*WSEG* = *19/19.0/36.1/12.9*)	DESCRIPTION OF THE ISSUE Should a doctor screen the vision of a patient over 65? (*WSEG* = *11/11.0/72.6/5.8*)
RECOMMENDATION The USPSTF concludes that the current evidence is insufficient to assess the balance of benefits and harms of screening for impaired visual acuity in older adults. (*WSEG* = *26/26.0/37.2/14.5*)	RECOMMENDATION (UPDATE) None. We don't think there is enough evidence to decide this. (*WSEG* = *11/5.5/ 85.8/2.6*)

[i]US Preventive Services Task Force, "Screening for Impaired Visual Acuity in Older Adults: US Preventive Services Task Force Recommendation Statement," *JAMA* 315, no. 9 (2016): 908.

We can make this statement clearer by revising it to state the issue in shorter, real-world terms. Getting the first step right, by stating the issue in real-world terms, helps make everything that follows easier to understand.

Though it's usually best to start a narrative by talking about the real world, there are a few exceptions. An article could start with a well-known abstract concept and move to more concrete discussion. For example, an article could start by taking about the theory of evolution, a well-known abstract concept, and go on to talk about how it applies in immune therapy used to treat a patient with HIV.

Exercise 9.B. Start by anchoring your discussion in the real world
Look again at the excerpt *Mathematical Modeling of Kidney Transport* in Appendix 2.

Does the narrative start by talking about the real world? Or does it seem abstract?

Compare your answer to the Exercise Key in Appendix 3.

C. Choose a good narrative pathway

If a good narrative starts with things known and in the real world, where should it go from there? The key is to pick a good narrative pathway, make it clear to the

Table 9-2. **Examples of common narrative pathways**

Size	Proceeds from big to small or vice versa.
List	A set of items that have something in common.
Time	Starts with earlier events and proceeds to later events.
Process	Actions in a particular order: step 1, step 2, etc.
Pyramid	Starts by describing general information and then gives more detailed information.
Problem/solution	Starts by describing a problem and then gives a solution.
Status quo/alternative/ difference	Starts by describing the status quo, tells what's wrong with the status quo, presents an alternative, and evaluates the difference.
Real world/abstract	Starts by describing real-world things or actions (e.g., data) and then moves to more abstract analysis.

reader, and stick to it. It often helps a reader follow a narrative if they know where it is going. Table 9-2 shows examples of common narrative pathways.

How can you make your narrative pathway clear to the reader? It often takes only a simple cue. Consider the paragraph heading: "How Common is Barrett Esophagus and What Are the Risk Factors?"[3] From this statement, the reader learns what types of information will follow. But a reader might be confused if this same paragraph went on to talk about the history of Barrett's Esophagus or ways to treat it.

Exercise 9.C. Choose a good narrative pathway
Look again at the first two paragraphs of the excerpt from *Mathematical Modeling of Kidney Transport* in Appendix 2.

1. What narrative pathways does the narrative follow?
2. Does it state them explicitly? Or are they clear from context?
3. Does the excerpt follow each narrative pathway consistently?

Compare your answers to the Exercise Key in Appendix 3.

D. Make a smooth transition between concrete and abstract

One big challenge of medical writing is to make a smooth transition between concrete and abstract, or vice versa. It is often a smooth and natural transition to move from the real world to abstract analysis. Most research articles have separate sections for *study design, patients* or *study subjects, study outcomes,* and *interpretation of results.* Within each section, it is often clear from context whether the discussion deals with the real world or abstract ideas. Keeping real-world and abstract ideas in separate sentences or paragraphs can also help make the transition clear.

Exercise 9.D. Make a smooth transition between concrete and abstract
Look again at the first two paragraphs of *Mathematical Modeling of Kidney Transport* in Appendix 2.

1. What real-world things and actions does the narrative mention? What abstract ideas does it mention? Does the narrative make a smooth transition between concrete and abstract?
2. In what way are a rat kidney and a human kidney enough alike that it makes sense to compare them? Does the narrative explain this?
3. In what way are the kidneys of a rat, human, elephant and whale enough alike we can generalize about an abstract "mammal kidney?" Does the narrative explain this?
4. Write a paragraph that tells why we can generalize about a "mammal kidney." Compare the number of nephrons in a rat kidney and a human kidney.

Conclusion

In this chapter, we talked about choosing a clear narrative pathway. This usually involves starting with things known and anchoring the discussion in the real world. From there, choose a good narrative pathway, make it clear to the reader, and stick to it. Make a smooth transition between concrete and abstract.

We develop these ideas further in the next chapter, where we give tips on forging a strong chain of logical reasoning.

Notes

1. Quoted in Williams, *Style: Lessons in Clarity,* 74 (see Preface, n. 8).
2. Bujamda, "Effect of Aspirin and," 683 (see chap. 1, n. 27).
3. Zimmerman, "Common Questions about Barrett's," 92 (see chap. 2, n. 16).

CHAPTER 10

Forge a strong chain of logical reasoning

Looking back, I think it was more difficult to see what the problems were than to solve them.—Charles Darwin[1]

Why doesn't an expert write clearly? In this chapter, we give the second part of our answer. An expert, someone "too close" to their subject, doesn't always present a strong chain of logical reasoning. Sometimes they leave out a step of reasoning that seems obvious to them or present ideas in a confusing order (Table 10-1).

Many subjects would interest a wider audience, if only the author would explain the subject step by step in the right order. In this chapter, we give tips on forging a strong chain of logical reasoning.

A. Explain each step of reasoning

A good narrative explains each step of reasoning. Somebody too close to their subject may skip a step of reasoning they think seems obvious. But what seems obvious to an expert may not be obvious to the widest reasonable audience. Nobody ever tries to skip a step of reasoning, but it happens. Peer review may not always catch a missing step, especially when the reviewer is an insider, and the article's reasoning is clouded by *medicus incomprehensibilis*.

How do you spot a missing step of reasoning? The best way is to write in plain English, so any gap in reasoning becomes easier to see and fix.

Exercise 10.A. Explain each step of reasoning
Look again at *Mathematical Modeling of Kidney Transport* in Appendix 2.

Table 10-1. **An expert often leaves out steps of reasoning**

They talk about...	*but fail to first explain...*
how to solve a problem	*what* the problem is or *why* it is important
the problem in abstract terms	the problem in real-world terms
details or steps of reasoning	things to be proven or conclusions
a formula or equation in symbols	the formula or equation in words

The narrative starts by talking about the major parts of a kidney, the cortex and medulla. It goes on to talk about a nephron and its parts.

1. Where is a nephron located in relation to the cortex and medulla?
2. Does the excerpt explain this? Or has it left out a step of reasoning?

Compare your answers to the Exercise Key in Appendix 3.

B. State the problem before you solve it

A medical research article often involves answering three questions: What? Why? and How?

WHAT?

What is the problem? What is the question the research project is designed to address? Most medical research sets out to answer a question (e.g., *Does treatment "A" work better than treatment "B?" Does the new medicine work better than the old one?*)

WHY?

Why is the question or problem important? For a doctor or other medical scientist, a problem becomes important when it affects the health or treatment of a patient.

HOW?

How did the research seek to answer the question or solve the problem? How was the experiment or trial conducted?

It can be harder to follow a narrative that mixes up these three questions or leaves one of them out. Some authors try to tell *what they did* and *how they did it* in the same sentence. Some explain *how* they solved a problem without first stating clearly, *what* the problem is, or *why* it is important. Some authors explain *how* they carried out their research without first clearly stating *what* the question was their research was designed to answer. A good statement of the research question or problem goes a long way toward helping a reader understand the solution.

A medical research article starts with an abstract that addresses the *what, why* and *how* questions. But an abstract doesn't always frame these questions as clearly as it might. For example, consider the statements of "Importance" and "Objective" from a research article abstract in Table 10-2.

Do these statements answer the *what* and *why* questions as clearly as possible? We can understand these statements with a little study. But we can revise to state the research question, and tell why it is important, more simply and clearly. No doubt the authors had to write their abstract to fit the journal's format, which required them to state their research "objective" rather than to frame the research question.

The main text also addresses the research question, but clouds it with details of research method and analysis.

> The primary objective of this trial was to determine whether degludec/liraglutide was noninferior to up-titration of glargine in change from

Table 10-2. **State the problem before you solve it**

Original[i]	Revised
Importance	Importance
Achieving glycemic control remains a challenge for patients with type 2 diabetes even with insulin therapy. (*wseg = 16/16.0/26.6/13.5*)	For a patient with type 2 diabetes, it can be hard to keep blood sugar under control, even if they take insulin. (*wseg = 22/22.0/65.2/9.6*)
Objective	Objective—Issue addressed
To assess whether a fixed ratio of insulin degludec/liraglutide was noninferior to continued titration of insulin glargine in patients with uncontrolled type 2 diabetes treated with insulin glargine and metformin. (*wseg = 31/31.0/3.4/20.4*)	A patient has type 2 diabetes. Their doctor treats them using insulin glargine and metformin. If this doesn't work to control their blood sugar, the common next step is to raise their insulin dose, as needed. This study poses the question: Would it work just as well to use a fixed ratio of insulin degludec/liraglutide? (*wseg = 56/14.0/67.2/7.3*)

[i]Lingvay I, et al. "Effect of Insulin Glargine Up-titration vs Insulin Degludec/Liraglutide on Glycated Hemoglobin Levels in Patients With Uncontrolled Type 2 Diabetes—The DUAL V Randomized Clinical Trial," *JAMA* 315, no. 9 (2016): 898.

baseline HbA$_{1c}$ level in patients with uncontrolled type 2 diabetes treated with glargine and metformin. If the primary objective was met, secondary objectives were to assess whether degludec/liraglutide was statistically superior compared with glargine in change from baseline of HbA$_{1c}$ level, body weight, and rate of confirmed hypoglycemia.[2] *(WSEG = 70/35.0/4.5/21.3)*

Part of what makes this excerpt hard to understand is that it covers both *what* (the research question) and *how* (research method and analysis). The research question is: *Does degludec/liraglutide work as well as insulin glargine with metformin to help control a patient's diabetes?*

The research method involves how the researchers designed the clinical trial, and analyzed the data, in order to answer the research question. This involves talk of: *up-titration, baseline HbA$_{1c}$ level, statistically superior, body weight,* and *rate of confirmed hypoglycemia.* The statement of the research question would be clearer if the discussion of *what* and *how* were kept separate.

Exercise 10.B.   State the problem before you solve it
Look again at *Mathematical Modeling of Kidney Transport* in Appendix 2.

1. What happens if a person's kidney stops filtering blood as it should?
2. Why is it important to have a math model of how the kidney filters blood?
3. Does the excerpt help you to answer these questions?

Compare your answers to the Exercise Key in Appendix 3.

C. Say it in words before you say it in symbols

Medical writing sometimes presents an equation or formula in symbols without ever saying, in words, what the equation or formula represents. Consider the equation, $2223 - (20 \times 60) = 1023$. Stated in symbols alone, it's impossible to see why this equation or its solution are important.

But if we state the problem in words, its importance becomes clear and vivid.

The HMS Titanic sailed on its maiden voyage in April 1912 with 2223 passengers and crew aboard. The ship had 20 lifeboats, and each lifeboat could carry 60 people. If the ship were to strike an iceberg and sink quickly, far from any source of help, how many people would have to be left behind?

Table 10-3. **Words and symbols help make a smooth transition**

Words	Words & symbols	Symbols
We need to prepare a field hospital to care for patients during a sudden Ebola outbreak in a remote location. One truck can carry seven tents, with eight cots for each tent. How many patients can we accommodate using each truckload of equipment?	7 tents × 8 cots =? patient capacity per truckload	$7 \times 8 = 56$

MAKING A SMOOTH TRANSITION

Stating a problem in words makes it vivid and easy to understand. Stating it in symbols makes it easy to solve. Using a combination of words and symbols can sometimes help make a smooth transition between the two. (Table 10-3)

A schematic diagram sometimes serves as an intermediate step between the real world and abstract analysis. Thus, it can help make a smooth transition. For example, it is common for a schematic diagram of the circulatory system to show a simplified drawing of the heart, veins and arteries. Arrows show the direction of blood flow. Areas where oxygenated blood flows are commonly colored in red. Areas where de-oxygenated blood flows are commonly colored in blue. As such, some aspects of the diagram depict the real-world, other aspects seem more like abstract ideas.

One common way to make a smooth transition is to state a problem three times: (1) once in real-world terms (in words), (2) again in terms of math or other scientific concepts (in words), and (3) a third time in math or other scientific symbols. Taking care to make a smooth transition can go a long way towards presenting a logical argument clearly.

For example, suppose a patient has hip surgery and the doctor wants to prescribe oral pain medicine for them. How does a doctor figure the right dose? A good description may involve stating the problem three times (Table 10-4).

In a journal, this narrative might look like this:

What is the right oral dose of medicine to relieve a patient's pain? It is the dose that achieves a concentration of medicine in the patient's plasma that is both safe and effective. This is called, the target therapeutic concentration (TTC). To be effective, the TTC needs to be higher than, or equal to, the minimum effective concentration (MEC). To be

Table 10-4. **Three ways to describe dosing for pain medicine**

Oral dose	Concentration in plasma	Math
What is the right oral dose of medicine to relieve a patient's pain?	It is the dose that achieves a concentration of medicine in the patient's plasma that is both safe and effective. This is called, the target therapeutic concentration (TTC). To be effective, the TTC needs to be higher than, or equal to, the minimum effective concentration (MEC). To be safe, the TTC needs to be lower than, or equal to, the maximum safe concentration (MSC).	We can express this idea in the equation: $MEC \le TTC \le MSC$.

safe, the TTC needs to be lower than, or equal to, the maximum safe concentration (MSC). We can express this idea in the equation: $MEC \le TTC \le MSC$.[3] *(WSEG = 88/14.6/65.0/7.8)*

Exercise 10.C. Say it in words before you say it in symbols
Look again at the excerpt from *Mathematical Modeling of Kidney Transport* in Appendix 2. The excerpt presents three equations.

1. Does the narrative tell in words what each equation represents?
2. Does it otherwise explain them well enough for the widest reasonable audience to understand?

Compare your answers to the Exercise Key in Appendix 3.

Conclusion

In this chapter, we gave tips to help you forge a strong chain of logical reasoning: Explain each step of reasoning. State the problem before you solve it. Say it in words before you say it in symbols.

Notes

1. Quoted in Williams, *Style: Lessons in Clarity*, 185 (see Preface, n. 8).
2. Lingvay I, et al. "Effect of Insulin Glargine Up-titration vs Insulin Degludec/Liraglutide on Glycated Hemoglobin Levels in Patients With Uncontrolled Type 2 Diabetes—The DUAL V Randomized Clinical Trial," *JAMA* 315, no. 9 (2016): 898–899.
3. Linares O, et al. "Personalized Oxycodone Dosing: Using Pharmacogenetic Testing and Clinical Pharmacokinetics to Reduce Toxicity Risk and Increase Effectiveness," *Pain Med* 15, no. 5 (2014).

Afterword—Can things ever change?

The formulation of a problem is often more essential than its solution, which may be merely a matter of mathematical or experimental skill. To raise new questions, new possibilities, to regard old questions from a new angle, requires creative imagination and marks real advance in science.—Albert Einstein

In the 21st century, English is the global language of medical science. Reaching the widest reasonable audience requires writing in a way that is understandable.

In this book, we showed how *medicus incomprehensibilis* mostly stems from needless grammatical complexity. We identified several over-used writing habits that are symptoms of this complexity. We showed how you can use a small collection of plain English writing tips to treat *medicus incomprehensibilis* and improve reading ease, vividness and logical flow.

Change comes when people share a vision. We hope this book has provided a clear vision of *what* plain English is, *why* it's important, and *how* to use it to improve your medical writing.

Appendix 1

ENGLISH SPEAKERS AROUND THE WORLD

Introduction

Anybody who wants to write for the widest reasonable audience needs to consider the world's non-native English speakers. This appendix surveys English speakers around the world, including both native and non-native speakers. We present data on English speakers in general, since it gives a rough idea of where the world's English-speaking doctors live.

Non-native English speakers constitute the majority of the world's total English speakers. In predominantly English-speaking countries, they are an important minority. Since doctors are among the best-educated people in any country, it stands to reason they are over-represented among each country's English speakers. For example, if 10% of India's citizens speak English, it stands to reason far more than 10% of Indian doctors speak English. (We think the number is closer to 100%.) The same probably holds true in any other country where learning English is considered part of a "good education."

What does it mean to be an "English speaker?"

The language skills of English speakers vary. A non-native speaker who has lived all their life in England may speak English better than most native speakers. Other non-native speakers may speak English well, but not as well as a native speaker. For example, a German doctor may have good scientific training and read and speak English well, but they might not speak English as well as a high-school graduate from Australia.

The world's top 25 English-speaking countries

Table A1-1 shows a list of the world's top 25 English speaking countries. More than half the world's population lives in these countries.

Table A1-1. World's top 25 English-speaking countries (population in millions)[i]

		Total Population (millions)	English Speakers (millions)	%	On which continent?					
					Asia	North America	Europe	Africa	Australia	South America
1	United States	317	298	94%		298				
2	India	1,210	125	10%	125					
3	Pakistan	188	92	49%	92					
4	Nigeria	156	83	53%				83		
5	UK	64	64	100%			64			
6	Philippines	100	64	64%	64					
7	Germany	81	52	64%			52			
8	Bangladesh	163	30	18%	30					
9	Canada	33	28	85%		28				
10	Egypt	83	28	34%				28		
11	France	65	26	40%			26			
12	Italy	60	20	33%			20			
13	Australia	21	17	81%					17	
14	Thailand	63	17	27%	17					
15	South Africa	53	16	30%				16		
16	Netherlands	17	15	89%			15			
17	Poland	39	14	37%			14			

#	Country									
18	Nepal	30	14	47%		14				
19	Turkey	71	12	17%		12				
20	Iraq	32	11	34%		11				
21	Brazil	205	11	5%						11
22	Spain	47	10	21%			10			
23	China	1,200	10	1%		10				
24	Sweden	10	8	81%			8			
25	Kenya	43	8	19%				8		
	Total	4,350	1,073	25%	375	326	209	135	17	11

¹We took data for Population and English Speakers from Wikipedia, s.v. "List of Countries by English-Speaking Population," https://en.wikipedia.org/wiki/List_of_countries_by_English-speaking_population (accessed May 5, 2016) and rounded to the nearest million. We figured % by dividing English Speakers by Population. We included Turkey in the Asia column, though partly in Europe.

English is strongly represented on every continent except South America and Antarctica. The list in Table A1-1 includes nine countries in Asia, eight in Europe, and four in Africa. Asia now has more English speakers than any other continent, and the number of English speakers there seems poised to grow in the future.

USA, UK, CANADA AND AUSTRALIA

These large countries, where most people speak English, are home to 407 million people or 5.5% of the world's population.[1] Within these countries, about 14% of the total population, or 59 million people, are non-native English speakers. Taken together, these countries have 247 medical schools (Table A1-2).

How many doctors in these countries are non-native English speakers? Fourteen percent? More, or fewer? We don't know, but we think the number is fairly high.

INDIA, PAKISTAN, NIGERIA, THE PHILIPPINES, BANGLADESH AND EGYPT

These six large countries with old colonial ties to the UK or USA are home to 1,900 million people, more than 25% of the world's population. In these

Table A1-2. **USA, UK, Canada, Australia—English speakers/medical schools[i]**

	Native		Non-native		Total	Medical
	(millions)	%	(millions)	%	(millions)	schools
USA[ii]	256	86%	43	14%	298	178
UK[iii]	59	92%	5	8%	64	31
Canada[iv]	19	68%	9	32%	28	17
Australia[v]	15	88%	2	12%	17	21
Total	349	86%	59	14%	407	247

[i]Population data, same source as Table A1-1.

[ii]USA "Medical schools" represent 145 accredited MD-granting institutions plus 33 accredited DO-granting institutions; American Association of Medical Colleges, "About the AAMC," (accessed May 12, 2016) https://www.aamc.org/about/; American Association of Colleges of Osteopathic Medicine, "U.S. Colleges of Osteopathic Medicine," (accessed May 12, 2016) http://www.aacom.org/become-a-doctor/us-coms.

[iii]UK General Medical Counsel, "Bodies Awarding UK Medical Degrees," (accessed May 12, 2016) http://www.gmc-uk.org/education/undergraduate/awarding_bodies.asp.

[iv]Association of Faculties of Medicine of Canada, "Accredited Canadian Medical Education Programs," (accessed May 12, 2016) https://www.afmc.ca/accreditation/committee-accreditation-canadian-medical-schools-cacms/accredited-canadian-medical.

[v]Australian Medical Council Ltd., "Accredited Medical Schools," (accessed May 12, 2016) http://www.amc.org.au/accreditation/primary-medical-education/schools.

countries, about 422 million people—about 22%—speak English. They have 676 medical schools (Table A1-3). In these countries, getting a "good education" includes learning English. We assume most doctors in these countries speak and read English well.

These countries have 4.7 times as many people and 2.7 times as many medical schools as the USA, UK, Canada and Australia combined. (Table A1-4). They have slightly more English speakers.

EUROPE

Europe is home to about 740 million people, or about 11% of the world's population.[2] European researchers publish widely in English-language journals. About 13% of Europeans speak English as a native language, mostly in the UK and Ireland. Another 38%, about 191 million, speak English as an additional language.[3]

Table A1-3. **India, Pakistan, Nigeria, The Philippines, Bangladesh, Egypt— English speakers/medical schools[i]**

| | English Speakers | | Total pop. | Medical |
	(millions)	%	(millions)	Schools
India[ii]	125	10%	1,210	398
Pakistan[iii]	92	49%	188	97
Nigeria[iv]	83	53%	156	27
Philippines[v]	64	64%	100	38
Bangladesh[vi]	30	18%	163	93
Egypt[vii]	28	34%	83	8
Total	422	22%	1,900	676

[i]Population data, same source as Table A1-1.

[ii]Medical Council of India, "List of Colleges Teaching MBBS," (accessed May 25, 2016) http://nri-educationalsociety.com/NRIACADEMYHOME/PDF/MCICOLLISTANDSEATS.PDF.

[iii]Pakistan Medical and Dental Council, "Recognized Medical Colleges In Pakistan," (accessed May 25, 2016) http://www.pmdc.org.pk/AboutUs/RecognizedMedicalDentalColleges/tabid/109/Default.aspx.; Schools no longer admitting students, and recommended for closure, have been excluded.

[iv]Nigeria Medical and Dental Council, "Accredited Medical Schools," (accessed May 12, 2016) https://www.mdcn.gov.ng/page/accredited-medical-schools; only fully accredited medical schools are counted.

[v]Association of Philippine Medical Colleges, "Member Schools and Colleges," http://www.apmcf-ph.net/member-schools-and-colleges.

[vi]Wikipedia, s.v. "List of medical colleges in Bangladesh" (accessed June 12, 2016) https://en.wikipedia.org/wiki/List_of_medical_colleges_in_Bangladesh.

[vii]Wikipedia, s.v. "List of Medical Schools in Egypt" (accessed May 12, 2016) https://en.wikipedia.org/wiki/List_of_medical_schools_in_Egypt.

Table A1-4. **Comparing large English-speaking countries**[i]

	USA, UK, Canada, Australia	India, Pakistan, Nigeria, The Philippines, Bangladesh, Egypt	Ratio
Total population (millions)	407	1900	1: 4.7
Percent of world population (%)	5.5%	25.6%	
English speakers	407	422	1: 1.04
Medical schools	247	676	1: 2.7

[i]Data from Tables A1-1 through A1-3.

English is the most widely spoken foreign language in the European Union. Overall, about 51% of the people of the European Union speak English.[4] This represents a total population four times the size of the UK. In some countries, a large majority of the people speak English, including the Netherlands (90%), Malta (89%), Sweden (86%), Cyprus (73%), Austria (73%) and Finland (70%).[5]

Based on this information, we know many European doctors read English-language medical journals. It also seems likely their level of medical science knowledge exceeds their level of English-language skills.

CHINA

In China, 10 million people speak English, less than 1% of the population. This number seems poised to grow in coming years, since China has another 300 million "learners."[6] If just 5% of these "learners" successfully learn English, it would add a new population of English speakers the size of the UK. (A 5% rate would be about the same as in Brazil, where relatively few people speak English.)

We assume English-language medical literacy in China is low. As more Chinese people learn English, we expect the number of Chinese doctors who read English language medical journals to grow even faster. Plain English medical writing would help to speed up this process.

Conclusion

Given the large and ever-increasing number of English speakers around the world, it makes sense to write about medical science in plain English. Many researchers write their articles in English, though English is not their native language. The data suggest non-native speakers now comprise a large part of the audience for English-language medical journals. More doctors would read English language journals, and understand them better, if they were written in plain English.

Notes

1. World population estimate of 7,429 million based on World Population Clock, (accessed June 13, 2016) http://www.worldometers.info/world-population/.
2. Wikipedia s.v. "Demographics of Europe," (accessed June 12, 2016) https://en.wikipedia.org/wiki/Demographics _of_Europe.
3. TNS Opinion & Social, *Europeans and Their Languages*, Special Eurobarometer 386 (Brussels: European Commission, June 2012), 5–6, 23.
4. Wikipedia, s.v. "Language in Europe," (accessed June 21, 2016) https://en.wikipedia.org/wiki/English_language_in _Europe.
5. TNS Opinion & Social, *Europeans and Their Languages*, Special Eurobarometer 386 (Brussels: European Commission, June 2012), 23.
6. Yang J, "Learners and users of English in China," *English Today* 22, no. 2 (April 2006): 3–10.

Appendix 2

SELECTED EXCERPTS FROM MEDICAL SCIENCE ARTICLES

1. Mathematical Modeling of Kidney Transport: Glomerular Filtration[1]

Most mammalian kidneys have three major sections: the cortex, the outer medulla, and the inner medulla. The outer and inner medulla are collectively referred to as the medulla. The outer medulla may be divided into the outer stripe and the inner stripe.

The functional unit of the kidney is the nephron; see Fig. 1. Each rat kidney (which is the most well-studied mammalian kidney) is populated by about 38,000 nephrons; each human kidney consists of about a million nephrons. Each nephron consists of an initial filtering component called the renal corpuscle and a renal tubule specialized for reabsorption and secretion. The renal corpuscle is composed of a glomerulus and the Bowman's capsule. A glomerulus is a tuft of capillaries arising from the afferent arterioles. Some of the water and solutes in the blood supplied by the afferent arteriole are driven by a pressure gradient into the space formed by the Bowman's capsule. The remainder of the blood flows into the efferent arteriole.

The most notable models of filtration of blood by glomerular capillaries are by Deen and coworkers. Most glomerular filtration models idealize the tortuous capillaries as a network of identical, parallel, rigid cylinders with homogeneous properties. Model equations typically consist of a system of coupled ODEs expressing fluid and solute conservation:

$$\frac{\partial}{\partial x}(QC_k) = -\frac{S}{L}J_k$$

$$\frac{\partial}{\partial x}(Q) = -\frac{S}{L}J_v$$

$$\frac{\partial}{\partial x}\left(QC_{pr}\right)=0$$

where Q denotes plasma flow rate, S and L denote the surface area and length of the capillary, J_v and J_k denote the fluid and solute fluxes, C_k denotes the total plasma concentration (free and bound states) of solute k, the subscript pr denotes protein, and x denotes the position along the capillary. Boundary conditions are given for Q, C_k, and C_{pr} at the afferent end of the capillary. Volume flux is assumed to be driven by hydrostatic and oncotic pressure differences, and fluxes for small solutes (smaller than proteins) are assumed to be both advective and diffusive, through the fenestrated capillary walls. *(WSEG = 320/20.0/41.4/11.8)*

2. The Frequency and Cost of Treatment Perceived to be Futile in Critical Care[2]

Advances in medicine enable critical care specialists to save lives as well as prolong dying. An admission to the intensive care unit (ICU) should be considered a therapeutic trial—aggressive critical care should transition to palliative care once it is clear that the treatment will not achieve an acceptable health state for the patient. However, intensive care interventions often sustain life under circumstances that will not achieve an outcome that patients can meaningfully appreciate. Such treatments are often perceived to be "futile" by health care providers. A survey of ICU physicians in Canada found that as many as 87% believe that futile treatment had been provided in their ICU in the past year. In a single-day cross-sectional study performed in Europe, 27% of ICU clinicians believe that they provided "inappropriate" care to at least 1 patient, and most of the inappropriate care was deemed such because it was excessive. *(WSEG = 149/24.8/37.9/14.1)*

3. Regulation of GPCRs by Endocytic Membrane Trafficking and its Potential Implications[3]

An essential requirement for maintenance of homeostasis in any living organism is the ability of cells to sense the external environment and, in the case of multicellular organisms, for cells to communicate with each other via mediators released into the extracellular milieu. Equally important are mechanisms for cells to rapidly adapt to changes in these extracellular signals, as evident in various disease processes characterized by uncontrolled or inadequately controlled cellular signaling. Accordingly, many important physiological processes are governed by the coordinated actions of multiple receptor-mediated signaling pathways, each of which is capable of rapid and specific regulation. Achieving this regulation is highly pertinent for G protein-coupled receptors (GPCRs), which represent the largest family of signaling receptors expressed in animals and respond to a wide range of stimuli. The diverse physiological roles served by GPCRs, together with evidence for disordered GPCR signaling in various pathological conditions, emphasize the fundamental biological and clinical importance of GPCRs, and support their prominent position as targets in drug development programs. *(WSEG = 166/33.2/0.0/22.7)*

Notes

1. Layton A, "Mathematical Modeling of Kidney Transport," *NIH Public Access*, under "2. Glomerular Filtration," http://www.ncbi.nlm.nih.gov/pmc/articles/PMC3745785/; originally published in *Wiley Interdiscip Rev Syst Bio Med* 5, no. 5 (September 2013).
2. Huynh T, et al. "The Frequency and Cost of Treatment Perceived to be Futile in Critical Care," *JAMA Intern Med* 173, no. 20 (2013): 1888.
3. Hanyaloglu A, von Zastrow M, "Regulation of GPCRs by Endocytic Membrane Trafficking and Its Potential Implications," *Annual Review of Pharmacology and Toxicology* 48 (2008): 538.

Appendix 3

EXERCISE KEY

Introduction

Exercise A. Widest reasonable audience
1. We think the widest reasonable audience includes doctors, physiologists, pharmacists, mathematicians, biologists, bio-medical engineers, bio-chemists, and others. It might include researchers and advanced students in these fields.
2. A mathematician or engineer probably needs more information on kidney anatomy. A doctor probably needs a better explanation of math and fluid dynamics. For example, what is an ODE? (An ordinary differential equation?) Why explain kidney anatomy any doctor knows, but not technical jargon related to fluid dynamics some doctors don't know (e.g., *afferent, efferent, advective, oncotic, diffusive, fenestrated*)?

Exercise B. How does sentence length affect reading ease?
1. Excerpt 1 uses the shortest sentences. Excerpt 3 uses the longest. (Table A3-1)

Table A3-1. **Average sentence length**

Article		Average Sentence Length
1	Mathematical Modeling for Kidney Transport	14
2	Futile Critical Care	24
3	Regulation of GPCR's	35

2. We find the first excerpt, "Mathematical Modeling for Kidney Transport," easiest to read. It uses shorter sentences and seems more concise than the others. The second excerpt, on "Futile Critical Care," uses longer sentences and seems "wordy." The third excerpt, "Regulation of GPCR's by Endocytic Membrane

Trafficking," is the hardest to read. The subject is very technical. It uses long sentences and many long words.

3. Yes, there seems to be a general correlation between reading ease and sentence length.

Exercise C. Recognizing symptoms of medicus incomprehensibilis
Table A3-2 identifies the symptoms of *medicus incomprehensibilis*.

Table A3-2. **Exercise C. Symptoms of** *medicus incomprehensibilis* **observed**

	Excerpt 1	*Excerpt 2*	*Excerpt 3*
Low reading ease	✓	✓	✓
long sentence (>25 words)	✓	✓	✓
run-on sentence		✓	✓
dependent clause		✓	✓
parenthetical statement	✓		
long word	✓	✓	✓
passive voice	✓	✓	✓
Abstraction	✓	✓	✓
abstract language	✓	✓	✓
nominalization	✓	✓	✓
formality	✓	✓	✓
plural subject	✓	✓	✓
obscure jargon	✓		✓

Concept 1. Take charge of your reading ease score

Exercise D. Take charge of your reading ease score

1. Given the <u>complexity</u> of the immune system, the <u>development</u> of an <u>individual</u> B cell is <u>unlikely</u> to follow a <u>predictable</u> and <u>well-executed</u> series of <u>decision</u> points whereby an <u>antigen-reactive</u> cell is expanded to a clone that produces a single <u>antibody</u>. A more <u>realistic</u> <u>perspective</u> is that their <u>development</u> depends on a series of <u>error-prone</u>, random <u>rearrangement</u> events and <u>mutations</u> whereby <u>specificity</u> for the <u>original</u> <u>antigen</u> is maintained (or not) by <u>selective</u> pressures. *(WSEG = 72/36.0/3.4/21.7)*

2. complexity → complex; development → develop; individual → any one; unlikely → not likely; predictable → can predict; well-executed → done well; decision → decide; antigen-reactive → reacts to an

antigen; more realistic perspective → more likely; error-prone → prone to error; rearrangement → re-arrange; mutations → mutate; specificity → specify; original → first; selective → select.

We consider *antibody* and *antigen* essential scientific terms.
Revision:

> 3. Given how complex the immune system is, any one B cell is not likely to <u>develop</u> in a way that is easy to predict. For example, a cell that reacts to an <u>antigen</u> expands to a clone that produces a single <u>antibody</u>. More likely, the cell <u>develops</u> through a series of <u>error-prone</u>, random events, in which it mutates and becomes re-arranged. In the process, <u>selective</u> pressures <u>determine</u> whether the cell still <u>specifies</u> the <u>original antigen</u>. *(WSEG = 75/18.7/52.4/10.6)*

We find the revision easier to read than the original.

SUMMARY

Comparing before and after WSEG scores, we see reading ease improves by 49.0 points and the grade level drops by 11.1 grades (Table A3-3).

Table A3-3. **Exercise D. WSEG scores**

	Original				Revision			
	Total words	Avg. words per sentence	Reading ease	Grade level	Total words	Avg. words per sentence	Reading ease	Grade level
	W	S	E	G	W	S	E	G
Scores	72	36.0	3.4	21.7	75	18.7	52.4	10.6
Change					3	−17.3	49.0	−11.1

Chapter 1. Use normal sentence length

Exercise 1.A. Keep sentence length 15 words average, 25 words maximum

1. But the physician's subsequent choice to designate the hospital discharge as against medical advice and pursue the formalized process associated with it (eg, specialized discharge forms) has no evidence-based utility for patient care, is not legally required, and has been shown to be associated with reduced willingness for the patient to return for future care. *(WSEG = 55/55.0/0.2/26.8)*

As the *WSEG* score shows, the original sentence has 55 words.
  Revision:

> **But a doctor should think twice before labeling a hospital discharge as "against medical advice" and pursuing the formal process associated with it (eg, special discharge forms). Why? Because it doesn't help patient care, it isn't legally required, and it makes the patient less willing to return for future care.** *(WSEG = 50/16.6/57.9/9.3)*

The revision has three sentences with 27, 1, and 22 words. The sentences have a total of 50 words and an average sentence length of 16.6.

> **2. Our Review will focus on advances in understanding of COPD and its risk factors, prevalence, and natural history since these Reviews were published, address some of the questions that still persist, and raise some of the issues that health-care planners will have to consider as the burden of COPD increases as the world's population ages.** *(WSEG = 55/55.0/20.2/24.0)*

Revision:

> **Our Review focuses on new knowledge of COPD and its risk factors, prevalence, and history since these Reviews were published. It addresses some questions that still persist. It also raises some issues health-care planners must think about as the burden of COPD increases as the world's people age.** *(WSEG = 48/16.0/61.9/8.5)*

> **3. Since *CYP2C9* explained 6 to 10 percent of the variability in these two patient samples, the *VKORC1* genotype appears to be the most important genetic factor determining variability in warfarin dose: in both clinical populations its effect was approximately three times that of the *CYP2C9* genotype.** *(WSEG = 46/46.0/1.9/24.4)*

Revision:

> ***CYP2C9* explains 6 to 10% of the variability in these two patient samples. The *VKORC1* genotype seems to be the key genetic factor that determines variability in warfarin dose. In both study groups, its effect was about three times that of the *CYP2C9* genotype.** *(WSEG = 44/14.6/53.5/9.4)*

> **4. A systematic review of randomized clinical trials of multiple risk factor interventions for preventing ischaemic heart disease had a modest effect on changes in lifestyle factors, cholesterol concentrations, and blood pressure—the last two mainly owing to**

the drug treatment used—but no significant effect on long term mortality due to ischaemic heart disease. *(WSEG = 54/54.0/0.0/27.3)*

Revision:

We reviewed randomized clinical trials of multiple risk factor interventions to prevent ischaemic heart disease. These interventions had a modest effect on lifestyle, cholesterol levels, and blood pressure. The last two were mainly owing to the drug treatment used. Over the long term, we found no significant effect on the death rate due to ischaemic heart disease. *(WSEG = 57/14.2/49.8/9.8)*

5. Over the past 100 years, the science of exercise has grown from seminal discoveries documenting the effects of exercise intensity on vascular control, heat production, oxygen requirement, and lactic acid dynamics—which led to Nobel Prizes in physiology or medicine in 1920 (August Krogh, Denmark) and 1922 (A.V. Hill, United Kingdom and Otto Meyerhof, Germany)—to our modern-day understanding that one's cardiorespiratory fitness (indexed by one's maximum rate of oxygen consumption) is among the most powerful predictors of morbidity and mortality. *(WSEG = 81/81.0/0.0/40.7)*

Revision:

Over the past 100 years, exercise science has grown. It began with work showing how exercise affects vascular control, heat production, oxygen need, and lactic acid dynamics. This led to a Nobel Prize in physiology or medicine for August Krogh of Denmark in 1920. It led to another one for A.V. Hill of the United Kingdom and Otto Meyerhof of Germany in 1922. Since then other studies have led to our modern knowledge of fitness. We now know fitness, measured by a person's peak rate of oxygen use, strongly predicts their chance of illness or death. *(WSEG = 96/16.0/53.1/9.8)*

6. In a prospective study in the Netherlands that followed more than 30,000 students 10 to 14 years of age for up to three years, annual scoliosis screening in addition to the usual biennial health checkup detected no cases of idiopathic scoliosis requiring surgery, and the authors concluded that additional annual scoliosis screening was not needed. *(WSEG = 55/55.0/0.0/ 28.6)*

Revision:

One prospective study in the Netherlands followed 30,000 students age 10 to 14 for up to three years. Each year, a student had a scoliosis screening. (This was on top of their usual health checkup every two years.) The extra screening found no cases of idiopathic scoliosis that required surgery. Based on this result, the authors found the extra scoliosis screening was not needed. *(WSEG = 64/ 12.8/51.0/9.3)*

SUMMARY

This exercise asked you to practice using normal sentence length and making other changes to improve reading ease. Table A3-4 summarizes the *WSEG* scores for the original sentences and our revisions. On average, reading ease improved by 50.8 points and grade level dropped 19.3.

Table A3-4. **Exercise 1.A. WSEG scores**

	Original				Revision			
	Total words	Avg. words per sentence	Reading ease	Grade level	Total words	Avg. words per sentence	Reading ease	Grade level
	W	S	E	G	W	S	E	G
1	55	55.0	0.2	26.8	50	16.6	57.9	9.3
2	55	55.0	20.2	24.0	48	16.0	61.9	8.5
3	46	46.0	1.9	24.4	44	14.6	53.5	9.4
4	54	54.0	0.0	27.3	57	14.2	49.8	9.8
5	81	81.0	0.0	40.7	96	16.0	53.1	9.8
6	55	55.0	0.0	28.6	64	12.8	51.0	9.3
Average	57.7	57.7	3.7	28.6	59.8	15.0	54.4	9.4
Change					2.2	−42.6	50.8	−19.3

Exercise 1.B. Keep the subject and verb close together in the first seven or eight words

1. Although SDM is well accepted in overtly value-laden clinical decisions such as prostate-specific antigen testing and mammography screening, the <u>principles</u> of SDM <u>apply</u> to a broad range of health care decisions, discharges against medical advice included. *(WSEG = 36/36.0/0.0/22.3)*

Only two words separate the subject and the verb, but they do not come within the first eight words.

Revision:

> The <u>values</u> of SDM <u>apply</u> to a broad range of health care choices. <u>They</u> <u>are</u> well-accepted in value-laden choices such as prostate-specific antigen testing and mammogram screening. <u>They</u> also <u>apply</u> to a discharge against medical advice. *(WSEG = 36/12.0/48.9/9.4)*

> 2. The only comprehensive <u>effort</u> to date to estimate summary measures of population health for the world, by cause, <u>is</u> the ongoing Global Burden of Diseases, Injuries, and Risk Factors (GBD) enterprise. *(WSEG = 31/31.0/28.0/17.0)*

Fourteen words separate the subject, *effort,* and the verb, *is.* The verb does not come in the first eight words.
   Revision:

> The Global Burden of Diseases, Injuries, and Risk Factors (GBD) <u>enterprise</u> <u>is</u> the only comprehensive effort to date to estimate, by cause, the summary measures of population health for the world. The <u>GBD</u> <u>is</u> ongoing. *(WSEG = 35/17.5/48.8/10.7)*

In this revision, no words separate the subjects and verbs. The long name, "*Global Burden of Diseases, Injuries, and Risk Factors (GBD),*" prevents us from putting the subject, *enterprise*, within the first eight words.

> 3. Although drug effect is a complex phenotype that depends on many factors, early and often dramatic <u>examples</u> involving succinylcholine and isoniazid <u>facilitated</u> acceptance of the fact that inheritance can have an important influence on the effect of a drug. *(WSEG = 39/39.0/2.3/22.6)*

Only four words separate the subject and the verb, but they do not appear within the first eight words.
   Revision:

> <u>Genes</u> <u>have</u> a large influence on the effect of a drug. Drug <u>effect</u> <u>is</u> a complex phenotype that depends on many factors. Early <u>examples</u> that involved succinylcholine and isoniazid <u>helped make</u> this fact clear. *(WSEG = 34/11.3/58.4/7.9)*

> 4. Transparent <u>reporting</u> of review methods and detailed <u>reporting</u> of the clinical and methodological characteristics of the included studies and their results <u>are</u> important to enable a reader to judge

the reliability of both the review and the individual studies and to
assess their relevance to clinical practice and the meaning of the
results reported in the review. *(WSEG = 57/57.0/0.0/28.7)*

Nineteen words separate the first subject, *reporting,* and the verb, *are.* Thirteen
words separate the second subject, *reporting,* and the verb, *are.* The verb does not
come in the first eight words.
    Revision:

> What <u>should</u> a <u>review</u> of a primary study <u>include</u>? <u>It</u> <u>should</u> clearly
> report review methods and include details on clinical methods. <u>This</u>
> <u>allows</u> the reader to judge how reliable the review and the study
> are, and to assess how relevant the study is to clinical practice. <u>This</u>
> also <u>helps</u> a reader understand the results reported in the review.
> *(WSEG = 58/14.5/55.0/9.1)*

In the revision, the subjects and verbs are close together.

> 5. Baseline demographic <u>characteristics</u> and the <u>distribution</u> of
> perioperative ARDS risk factors or modifiers among those who did
> and did not develop postoperative ARDS (first procedure only) after
> bleomycin therapy <u>are presented</u> in table 2. *(WSEG = 34/34.0/0.0/
> 23.6)*

    Twenty-six words separate the first subject, *characteristics,* and the verb, *are
presented.* Twenty-three words separate the second subject, *distribution,* and the
verb, *are presented.* The verb does not come in the first eight words.
    Revision:

> <u>Table 2</u> <u>shows</u> demographic data and pre- and post- surgery ARDS
> risk factors. <u>It</u> <u>compares</u> data for those who did and did not have
> post-surgery ARDS after treatment with bleomycin. (First surgery
> only.) *(WSEG = 33/11.0/57.2/8.0)*

> 6. Because patients often are reluctant to discuss traumatic
> events and may avoid treatment as a result, <u>it</u> <u>is</u> important to
> elicit patient preferences for treatment interventions. *(WSEG =
> 26/ 26.0/21.0/16.7)*

In this example, the subject and verb are together, but they don't come within the
first eight words of the sentence.

Revision:

> **Some <u>patients</u> <u>don't want</u> to talk about a traumatic event, and may avoid treatment as a result. <u>That's</u> why it's important to talk with them about their preferences for treatment.** *(WSEG= 30/15.0/67.5/7.5)*

In the revision, no words separate the subjects and verbs.

SUMMARY

This exercise asked you to practice keeping the subject and the verb close together in the first seven or eight words. Table A3-5 shows the WSEG scores for our revisions.

Table A3-5. **Exercise 1.B. WSEG scores**

	Original				Revision			
	Total words	Avg. words per sentence	Reading ease	Grade level	Total words	Avg. words per sentence	Reading ease	Grade level
	W	S	E	G	W	S	E	G
1	36	36.0	0.0	22.3	36	12.0	48.9	9.4
2	31	31.0	28.0	17.0	35	17.5	48.8	10.7
3	39	39.0	2.3	22.6	34	11.3	58.4	7.9
4	57	57.0	0.0	28.7	58	14.5	55.0	9.1
5	34	34.0	0.0	23.6	33	11.0	57.2	8.0
6	26	26.0	21.0	16.7	30	15.0	67.5	7.5
Average	37.2	37.2	8.6	21.8	37.7	13.6	56.0	8.8
Change					0.5	−23.6	47.4	−13.1

Exercise 1.C. Put the main point first and then give commentary, detail or support

> 1. **Although Ontario surgeons receive a premium and bill accurately when they operate urgently between 12 AM and 7 AM, <u>the times and length of the overnight procedure and</u> also <u>how fatigued the surgeon truly was</u> when starting elective cases the next day <u>were unknown</u>.** *(WSEG = 44/44.0/16.0/21.9)*

Seventeen words come before the main point.
   Revision:

> We <u>don't know the time or length of the overnight procedure</u>. <u>We also don't know how tired each surgeon was</u> when they started the elective case the next day. We do know Ontario surgeons receive a premium when they operate urgently between 12 AM and 7 AM. They also bill accurately. *(WSEG = 51/12.7/62.8/7.6)*

> 2. First, <u>estimates</u> for 2000 <u>of</u> under-5 <u>mortality</u>, measured as the probability of death between 0 years and 5 years of age ($_5q_0$), and <u>mortality</u> as a young adult or middle-aged adult, measured as the probability of death between 15 years and 60 years of age ($_{45}q_{15}$), <u>were developed</u> after review of available vital registration, sample registration, and census data and the application of the synthetic extinct generation and growth balance methods to correct for under-registration of deaths. *(WSEG = 77/77.0/0.0/36.6)*

We think the main point is "estimates of . . . mortality. . . . were developed." You need to read the first 47 words before you can get the whole idea.
   Revision:

> <u>Our first task was to estimate mortality</u> for certain age ranges for the year 2000. We started by reviewing data we had on births, deaths and census. Then we corrected for under-reported deaths using the *synthetic extinct generation* and *growth balance* methods. We assessed under-5 mortality or $_5q_0$, and age 15-to-60 mortality or $_{45}q_{15}$. We defined "under-5 mortality" as "the chance of death between 0 and 5 years of age." We defined "age 15 to 60 mortality" as "the chance of death between 15 and 60 years of age." *(WSEG = 89/14.8/52.0/9.6)*

> 3. The trial showed that <u>pharmacogenetic-guided initiation of warfarin therapy resulted in a greater percentage of time in the therapeutic range, fewer excessive INRs, a shorter median time to therapeutic INR, and fewer dose adjustments</u>. *(WSEG = 34/34.0/0.6/21.6)*

This sentence already puts the main point first. But we can make it more concise, and move the supporting details to a second sentence.
   Revision:

> <u>The trial shows the benefits of starting warfarin treatment guided by a pharmacogenetic model</u>. They include more time in the

therapeutic range, fewer excess INRs, a shorter time to therapeutic INR, and fewer dose changes. *(WSEG = 35/17.5/41.6/11.8)*

4. <u>The participation rate was lower than we expected</u> when we did the power calculations; however, taking into account the fact that more people than expected had an increased risk and received counselling and that not even a trend to a reduction in ischaemic heart disease was observed, <u>we doubt that a participation rate of 70% would have made any difference</u>. *(WSEG = 60/60.0/38.2/15.3)*

We think there are two key points. One comes at the start, the other, 47 words into the sentence. We revised to put each key point at the start of its own sentence.

Revision:

<u>The participation rate was lower than we planned</u> when we did the power calculations. But <u>we doubt that a participation rate of 70% would have made any difference</u>. Though more people than expected had increased risk and received counselling, we saw no trend towards a decrease in ischaemic heart disease. *(WSEG = 50/16.6/56.2/9.5)*

5. <u>Recommended CRC screening strategies fall in 2 broad categories</u>: <u>stool tests</u> that primarily detect cancer, which include detection of occult blood or exfoliated DNA, <u>and structural tests</u>, such as flexible sigmoidoscopy, colonoscopy, and computed tomographic colonography, which are effective in detecting both cancer and premalignant lesions. *(WSEG = 46/46.0/0.0/27.4)*

This sentence spreads out the main point. You need to read 27 words to get the whole thing.

Revision:

<u>The recommended CRC screening tests fall in 2 broad classes: stool tests and structure tests</u>. A stool test mainly detects cancer by finding occult blood or fragments of DNA the body sheds in feces. A structure test helps detect cancer or a lesion in the colon that has not yet turned malignant. Some structure tests are: flexible sigmoidoscopy, colonoscopy, and CT colonography. *(WSEG = 62/15.5/58.7/8.9)*

6. According to the AUA, the presence of <u>three or more red blood cells on a single</u>, properly collected, noncontaminated <u>urinalysis</u> without evidence of infection <u>is considered clinically significant microscopic hematuria</u>. *(WSEG = 30/30.0/0.0/22.8)*

We think the main point is broken up throughout the sentence. You don't get the whole main point until the end. In the revision, we broke up this long sentence to make a short paragraph.

Revision:

> **When is microscopic hematuria "clinically significant?"** According to the AUA, **when a single urine test shows three or more red blood cells**. The urine sample must be collected in the right way, not contaminated, and show no sign of infection. *(WSEG = 40/ 13.3/49.4/9.6)*

SUMMARY

This exercise asked you to practice putting the main point first before giving commentary, detail or support. Table A3-6 shows the *WSEG* scores for our revisions.

Table A3-6. **Exercise 1.C. WSEG scores**

	Original				Revision			
	Total words	Avg. words per sentence	Reading ease	Grade level	Total words	Avg. words per sentence	Reading ease	Grade level
	W	S	E	G	W	S	E	G
1	44	44	16	21.9	51	12.7	62.8	7.6
2	77	77	0.0	36.6	89	14.8	52.0	9.6
3	34	34	0.6	21.6	35	17.5	41.6	11.8
4	60	60	38.2	15.3	50	16.6	56.2	9.5
5	46	46	0.0	27.4	62	15.5	58.7	8.9
6	30	30	0.0	22.8	40	13.3	49.4	9.6
Average	48.5	48.5	9.1	24.3	54.5	15.1	53.5	9.5
Change					6.0	−33.4	44.3	−14.8

Chapter 2. Prefer the short word

Exercise 2.A. Keep essential scientific terms; minimize other long words

1. Therefore, it is not <u>possible</u> to <u>determine</u> whether all <u>drug-eluting</u> stents could <u>benefit</u> from short-term <u>regimens</u> of dual <u>anti-platelet</u> <u>therapy</u> based on the <u>previous</u> trials reported. *(WSEG = 26/ 26.0/11.2/18.1)*

Revision:

Therefore, there is no way to tell if a <u>drug-eluting</u> stent could <u>benefit</u> from a short term course of dual <u>anti-platelet</u> treatment. We say this based on the prior trials reported. *(WSEG = 31/15.5/62.8/8.3)*

2. A careful <u>assessment</u> of the <u>demographic</u> <u>evidence</u> on the levels of <u>age-specific</u> <u>mortality</u> is an <u>integral</u> <u>component</u> of any Global Burden of Disease Study: such <u>analyses</u> require the sum of deaths from <u>specific</u> causes to equal the <u>independently</u> assessed level of <u>mortality</u> from all causes, for every age and sex group. *(WSEG = 51/51.0/0.0/26.7)*

Revision:

Any Global Burden of Disease Study must assess data with care. In this <u>assessment</u>, the sum of deaths by <u>specific</u> cause, age and sex must equal the sum of deaths from all causes assessed <u>separately</u>. *(WSEG = 35/17.5/63.3/8.7)*

3. Most of the <u>pharmacogenetic</u> traits that were first <u>identified</u> were <u>monogenic</u>—that is, they involved only a single gene—and most were due to <u>genetic</u> <u>polymorphisms</u>; in other words, the allele or alleles <u>responsible</u> for the <u>variation</u> were <u>relatively</u> common. *(WSEG = 40/40.0/34.2/13.4)*

Revision:

Most <u>pharmacogenetic</u> traits first <u>identified</u> involved only one gene. Most of these traits were due to <u>genetic</u> <u>polymorphism</u>. In other words, the allele or alleles that caused the <u>variation</u> were fairly common. *(WSEG = 32/10.6/50.6/8.8)*

4. <u>Diagnostic</u> <u>accuracy</u> is <u>essential</u> for good <u>therapeutic</u> treatment. *(WSEG = 8/8.0/0.0/17.0)*

Revision:

For a patient to get good treatment, the doctor needs to make the right <u>diagnosis</u>. *(WSEG = 15/15.0/73.1/6.7)*

5. The 2 <u>objectives</u> of the study were (1) to <u>examine</u> the <u>association</u> between <u>physical</u> <u>activity</u> and <u>dietary</u> <u>behavior</u> and (2) to <u>examine</u> the <u>potential</u> combined effect of <u>physical</u> <u>activity</u> and <u>dietary</u> <u>behavior</u> on <u>biological</u> (eg, total <u>cholesterol</u>) and health (eg, waist <u>circumference</u>) markers. *(WSEG = 43/43.0/0.0/25.8)*

Revision:

> **Our study checked the link between diet and exercise, and their combined effect on bio- and health- markers (eg, total <u>cholesterol</u> and waistline.)** *(WSEG = 23/23.0/51.0/11.8)*

6. **Assuming vasal <u>disruption</u> and <u>occlusion</u> have been <u>adequately</u> achieved during <u>surgery</u>, and assuming the patient adheres to using <u>another</u> <u>contraceptive</u> method while awaiting <u>confirmation</u> of <u>sterility</u>, true causes of <u>vasectomy</u> failure include <u>recanalization</u> (early and late) and, more rarely, <u>aberrant</u> <u>anatomy</u> (e.g., the presence of a third vas).** *(WSEG = 48/48.0/0.0/27.7)*

Revision:

> **Why does a <u>vasectomy</u> fail? The <u>surgery</u> may fail to disrupt and occlude the vas. A patient may fail to use other birth control while he waits for test results to prove he is sterile. The vas may <u>re-canalize</u> sooner or later. Or a patient may have odd <u>anatomy</u>, such as a third vas.** *(WSEG = 54/10.8/78.3/5.0)*

SUMMARY

This exercise asked you to keep essential scientific terms but minimize other long words. Table A3-7 shows the WSEG scores for our revisions.

Table A3-7. **Exercise 2.A. WSEG scores**

	Original				Revision			
	Total words	Avg. words per sentence	Reading ease	Grade level	Total words	Avg. words per sentence	Reading ease	Grade level
	W	S	E	G	W	S	E	G
1	26	26.0	11.2	18.1	31	15.5	62.8	8.3
2	51	51.0	0.0	26.7	35	17.5	63.3	8.7
3	40	40.0	34.2	13.4	32	10.6	50.6	8.8
4	8	8.0	0.0	17.0	15	15.0	73.1	6.7
5	43	43.0	0.0	25.8	23	23.0	51.0	11.8
6	48	48.0	0.0	27.7	54	10.8	78.3	5.0
Average	36.0	36.0	7.6	21.5	31.7	15.4	63.2	8.2
Change					−4.3	−20.6	55.6	−13.2

*Exercise 2.C. Write a compound word to promote reading ease and
show how you pronounce it*

    1. <u>Predefining</u> a threshold value for heart rate is difficult because it
must be individualized in the context of the patient's overall <u>hemo-
dynamic</u> status and any <u>preexisting</u> <u>comorbidities</u>. (WSEG = *27/27.0/
7.0/18.9*)

Pre-defining, pre-existing, hemo-dynamic, co-morbidity.
    Revision:

        It is not easy to <u>pre-define</u> a threshold value for heart rate. Any
        threshold must be set in the context of the patient's overall blood
        flow dynamics and any other <u>pre-existing</u> illness. (WSEG = *32/16.0/
        55.7/9.4)*

        2. For example, results of the Burden of Lung Disease (BOLD)
        study—a <u>multinational</u> investigation of the <u>prevalence</u> of COPD
        using a standard methodology and reported in this issue of *The
        Lancet*, show that one of the highest <u>prevalences</u> of COPD was
        recorded in South Africa, a country that also has a high <u>prevalence</u>
        of tuberculosis. (WSEG = *55/55.0/3.3/26.4)*

Multi-national. We wouldn't hyphenate *prevalence,* since it meets the three tests.
    Revision:

        This issue of *The Lancet* reports on the Burden of Lung Disease
        (BOLD) study. This study checked the number of cases of COPD in
        several countries using a standard method. It shows South Africa
        had one of the highest numbers. South Africa also had many cases
        of tuberculosis. (WSEG = *48/12.0/60.7/7.7)*

        3. Although a recent study showed that <u>genotype</u>-guided dosing
        led to superior control of <u>anticoagulation</u>, the finding was based
        on a comparison with a <u>nonrandomized</u>, real-world parallel control
        group. (WSEG = *28/28.0/6.1/19.3)*

Anti-coagulation and *non-randomized.* We wouldn't hyphenate *genotype* since it
meets the three tests and qualifies as an essential scientific term.
    Revision:

        One new study shows dosing guided by <u>genotype</u> gives better con-
        trol of <u>anti-coagulation.</u> But this finding was based on comparing

it to a <u>non-randomized</u>, real-world control group. (*WSEG =27/13.5/ 45.8/10.2*)

4. Flavonoids are naturally occurring <u>bioactive</u> compounds that represent a constituent of fruits and vegetables, beyond calorie and <u>macronutrient</u> content, that could potentially influence body weight. (*WSEG = 25/25.0/0.0/19.6*)

Bio-active, macro-nutrient.
  Revision:

Flavonoids are compounds found in fruits and vegetables. They may affect a person's body weight. This effect goes beyond calories and major nutrients. (*WSEG = 23/7.6/59.2/6.8*)

5. One of the identified causes of delay in ET is <u>multimodal</u> imaging. (*WSEG = 12/12.0/39.5/10.7*)

Multi-modal.
  Revision:

One cause of delay in ET is <u>multi-modal</u> imaging. (*WSEG = 9/9.0/ 56.7/7.5*)

6. The recommended modalities are <u>photodynamic</u> therapy, <u>radio-frequency</u> ablation, or <u>endoscopic</u> mucosal <u>resection</u>. (*WSEG = 12/ 12.0/0.0/26.4*)

Photo-dynamic. Radio frequency ablation is clear without a hyphen. We wouldn't hyphenate *endoscope*, the name of a common medical instrument. *Resection* meets the three tests.
  Revision:

The recommended treatments are <u>photo-dynamic</u> therapy, <u>radio frequency</u> ablation, or mucosal <u>resection</u> by <u>endoscope</u>. (*WSEG = 14/ 14.0/0.0/20.2*)

SUMMARY

This exercise asked you to practice writing a compound word to maximize reading ease and show how you pronounce it. Table A3-8 shows the WSEG scores for our revisions.

Table A3-8. **Exercise 2.C. WSEG scores**

	Original				Revision			
	Total words	Avg. Words per Sentence	Reading Ease	Grade Level	Total Words	Avg. Words per Sentence	Reading Ease	Grade Level
	W	S	E	G	W	S	E	G
1	27	27.0	7.0	18.9	32	16.0	55.7	9.4
2	55	55.0	3.3	26.4	48	12.0	60.7	7.7
3	28	28.0	6.1	19.3	27	13.5	45.8	10.2
4	25	25.0	0.0	19.6	23	7.6	59.2	6.8
5	12	12.0	39.5	10.7	9	9.0	56.7	7.5
6	12	12.0	0.0	26.4	14	14.0	0.0	20.2
Average	26.5	26.5	9.3	20.2	25.5	12.0	46.4	10.3
Change					−1.0	−14.5	37.0	−9.9

Exercise 2.D. Omit any unnecessary word ending

1. **Given that this was an observ<u>ational</u> study, unmeasured confounding or hidden bias might exist.** *(WSEG = 14/14.0/29.4/12.6)*

We thought *observational study* might qualify as an essential scientific term.
Revision:

Since this was an observ<u>ational</u> study, there might be unmeasured confounding or hidden bias. *(WSEG = 14/14.0/41.5/10.9)*

2. **However, poverty is regarded as a surrogate measure for many factors that subsequently increase the risk of COPD, such as poor nutrition<u>al</u> status, crowding, exposure to pollut<u>ants</u> including high work exposures and high smoking rates (in countries of low and middle income), poor access to health care, and early respirat<u>ory</u> infections.** *(WSEG = 51/51.0/4.1/25.3)*

We think *poor nutrition* or *poor nutrition status* works without the *–al* ending. You can also say *polluted air* rather than *pollutants*. We replaced *respiratory* with *lung*.
Revision:

But being poor is a proxy for factors that raise the risk for COPD. Poor people tend to live in crowded quarters with poor nutrition and poor access to health care. They breathe polluted air at work.

In low and middle income countries, many tend to smoke. All this helps cause early lung infection. *(WSEG = 54/10.8/84.6/4.1)*

3. The concept of pharmacogenetics originated from the clinical observation that there were patients with very high or very low plasma or urinary drug concentrations, followed by the realization that the biochemical traits leading to this variation were inherited. *(WSEG = 38/8.0/0.0/23.4)*

We think *urine drug concentration* is good modern English. The words, *clinical*, and *chemical* are used in common speech. But in the revision, we revised to avoid using *biochemical*.

Revision:

The concept of pharmacogenetics arose from clinical insight. Some patients had a very high or a very low concentration of a drug in their blood or urine. Doctors realized this was caused by the patient's genes. *(WSEG = 36/12.0/63.0/7.4)*

4. Benefit from combined mammography and breast physical examination screening was found in women aged 50–64, but not in women aged 40–49. *(WSEG = 21/21.0/4.2/17.8)*

We think *exam* and *mammogram* are good modern English. We would say, *age 50–64.*

Revision:

We found a benefit from combined mammogram and breast physical exam for women age 50 to 64. But we found none for women age 40 to 49. *(WSEG = 27/13.5/58.3/8.4)*

5. If familial cardiomyopathy is suggested on the basis of history, genetic testing and referral to a genetic counselor should be considered. *(WSEG = 21/21.0/4.2/17.8)*

The ending, *familial* is unnecessary, since you can just say, *family history of.* We think *gene testing* or *gene counselor* would sound awkward. *Referral* is plain English, but *refer* is shorter.

Revision:

What if the patient has a family history of heart muscle disease? In such cases, it is often best to refer them for genetic testing and counseling. *(WSEG = 27/13.5/61.5/8.0)*

6. Dosing must be tailored to the patient's symptoms and inflammatory markers because up to 13% of patients required higher initial doses. *(WSEG = 21/21.0/32.4/13.9)*

Both *inflammatory markers* and *inflammation markers* are used in scientific presentations.
Revision:

A doctor should tailor dosing to the patient's symptoms and inflammation markers. Up to 13% of patients may need a higher initial dose. *(WSEG = 23/11.5/59.0/7.8)*

SUMMARY

This exercise asked you to practice dropping any unneeded word ending. Table A3-9 shows the *WSEG* scores for our revisions.

Table A3-9. **Exercise 2.D. WSEG scores**

	Original				Revision			
	Total words	Avg. words per sentence	Reading ease	Grade level	Total words	Avg. words per sentence	Reading ease	Grade level
	W	S	E	G	W	S	E	G
1	14	14.0	29.4	12.6	14	14.0	41.5	10.9
2	51	51.0	4.1	25.3	54	10.8	84.6	4.1
3	38	38.0	0.0	23.4	36	12.0	63.0	7.4
4	21	21.0	4.2	17.8	27	13.5	58.3	8.4
5	21	21.0	4.2	17.8	27	13.5	61.5	8.0
6	21	21.0	32.4	13.9	23	11.5	59.0	7.8
Average	23	23.2	13	18	30	12.6	61.3	7.8
Change					7.0	−10.7	48.0	−9.9

Exercise 2.E. Avoid the noun string

1. The study by Vinden et al provides direct evidence from patient outcomes that operating the night before is not associated with

increased complications for <u>elective laparoscopic cholecystectomies</u> performed the following day. *(WSEG = 31/31.0/0.7/20.8)*

Revision:

The study by Vinden et al gives proof from patient outcomes. Operating the night before does not lead to more complications for elective laparoscopy to remove a gall bladder the next day. *(WSEG = 32/16.0/55.7/9.4)*

2. Performance is assessed in terms of <u>rigorous out-of-sample predictive validity testing</u> based on the <u>root-mean-squared error</u> of the log of the <u>age-specific death rates</u>, the percentage of time that trend is accurately predicted, and the coverage of the uncertainty intervals (UIs). *(WSEG = 41/41.0/8.4/22.2)*

Revision:

Through rigorous testing, we assessed how well each model performed. We tested how well the model predicts by using data from the sample. We checked the death rate for specific age groups using the <u>root-mean-square error</u> of the log. We checked how often the model accurately predicted a trend. We checked the coverage of the uncertainty intervals (UIs). *(WSEG = 58/11.6/63.7/7.2)*

We kept *root-mean-square error*, a standard statistical term.

3. By targeting VKOR, the <u>post-translational modification</u> of the <u>vitamin K-dependent blood-coagulation proteins</u> is impaired. *(WSEG = 14/14.0/0.0/18.5)*

Revision:

Targeting VKOR impairs the synthesis of proteins that use vitamin K to cause blood to coagulate. *(WSEG = 16/16.0/58.4/9.0)*

4. All participants with an unhealthy lifestyle had <u>individually tailored lifestyle counselling</u> at all visits (at baseline and after one and three years); those at high risk of ischaemic heart disease, according to predefined criteria, were furthermore offered six sessions of

group based lifestyle counselling on smoking cessation, diet, and physical activity. *(WSEG = 51/51.0/20.0/16.7)*

Revision:

Each person with an unhealthy lifestyle had one-on-one counselling. The counselling took place at each visit, starting at baseline and after one and three years. Each person with a high risk of ischaemic heart disease, as determined by fixed standards, was offered six sessions of group counselling. This counselling covered how to quit smoking, diet, and exercise. *(WSEG = 57/14.2/57.3/8.8)*

5. As in the original CMS readmission model derivation, patients who were discharged and then died before being rehospitalized were not counted as "failures"; that is, they were included in the analysis but not assigned a readmission event. *(WSEG = 37/37.0/ 41.7/12.0)*

Revision:

As with the original CMS model, we didn't count, as a "failure," a patient who was discharged, but then died without ever being rehospitalized. We included them in the analysis, but never counted them as re-admitted. *(WSEG = 36/18.0/56.0/8.4)*

6. Tick paralysis, which results from gravid female bites, is a toxin-mediated ascending paralysis that general resolves after tick removal. *(WSEG = 19/19.0/4.9/17.2)*

Revision:

Tick paralysis results from the bite of a pregnant female tick. Tick paralysis is a kind of ascending paralysis caused by a toxin. It generally resolves after the tick is removed. *(WSEG = 31/10.3/54.4/8.2)*

SUMMARY

This exercise asked you to practice identifying and eliminating noun strings. Table A3-10 shows the WSEG scores for our revisions.

Table A3-10. **Exercise 2.E. wseg scores**

	Original				Revision			
	Total words	Avg. words per sentence	Reading ease	Grade level	Total words	Avg. words per sentence	Reading ease	Grade level
	W	S	E	G	W	S	E	G
1	31	31.0	0.7	20.8	32	16.0	55.7	9.4
2	41	41.0	8.4	22.2	58	11.6	63.7	7.2
3	14	14.0	0.0	18.5	16	16.0	58.4	9.0
4	51	51.0	20.0	16.7	57	14.2	57.3	8.8
5	37	37.0	41.7	12.0	36	18.0	56.0	8.4
6	19	19.0	4.9	17.2	31	10.3	54.4	8.2
Average	32.2	32.2	12.6	17.9	38.3	14.4	57.6	8.5
Change					6.2	−17.8	45.0	−9.4

Exercise 2.F. Don't be afraid to start a sentence with and *or* but

1. Because patients with sepsis have a wide range of sympathetic activation and responsiveness, giving a fixed dose of a β-blocker would probably be less effective and potentially harmful if given to all patients. <u>Furthermore</u>, because adrenergic stress persists as long as the external stress (eg, infection or injury), treatment was continued for the entire intensive care unit stay. *(wseg = 58/29.0/ 27.1/16.6)*

We think "and" sounds okay. In our revision, we didn't use any conjunction to replace *furthermore*. We did use the conjunction *therefore* as a way to break up the long sentences.

Revision:

A patient with sepsis can have a wide range of sympathetic activation and response. Therefore, giving a fixed dose of a β-blocker is probably less effective and might also harm some patients. Adrenergic stress goes on as long as the external stress from illness or injury goes on. Therefore, we kept treating the patient for their whole ICU stay. *(wseg = 59/14.7/61.3/8.3)*

2. The period since 1970 has been characterized by substantial heterogeneity in mortality transitions. Life expectancy in Japanese women in 2010 was 85.9 years, and is probably higher in 2012.

However, the gain in the past 40 years was only 11 years, compared with total improvements of two to three times more in other parts of Asia (eg, the Maldives), the Middle East (especially Oman), and Latin American (eg, Bolivia, Peru, and Guatemala). *(WSEG = 72/24.0/ 17.9/16.7)*

We think "but" sounds okay.
  Revision:

Since 1970, the mean life span has changed unevenly. In 2010, a woman in Japan could expect to live 85.9 years and likely still longer in 2012. **But** the gain in the past 40 years was only 11 years. The gain was two to three times more in other parts of Asia (eg, the Maldives), the Middle East (eg, Oman), and Latin America (eg, Bolivia, Peru, and Guatemala). *(WSEG = 68/17.0/55.2/9.7)*

3. Our analysis does not address the issue of whether a precise initial dose of warfarin translates into improved clinical end points, such as a reduction in the time needed to achieve a stable therapeutic INR, fewer INRs that are out of range, and a reduced incidence of bleeding or thromboembolic events. **However**, our study lays important groundwork for a prospective trial and suggests that such a trial should be powered to detect the benefits of incorporating pharmacogenetic information into the dose algorithm for patients who require high or low doses—the subgroups in our study for whom dose estimates based on the pharmacogenetic algorithm differed significantly from those based on the clinical algorithm. *(WSEG = 113/56.5/0.5/27.2)*

These two long sentences draw a contrast between what the *analysis does not address* and what it *lays the groundwork for*. We think just inserting the word *but* would sound awkward since the contrasting ideas are so remote from each other. We re-phrased to put these ideas closer together, and used *but* in the middle of the sentence.
  Revision:

Does a precise starting dose of warfarin give a better clinical result? Does it help reduce the time needed to reach a stable therapeutic INR? Does it mean fewer INRs out of range? Does it reduce bleeding or thrombo-embolic events? Our study doesn't address these issues, **but** it does lay important groundwork for a future trial. The trial should be set up to detect the benefits of using pharmacogenetic data in the dose algorithm for a patient who needs a high or low dose. These were the groups in our study for whom the pharmacogenetic algorithm and the clinical algorithm gave significantly different dose estimates. *(WSEG = 105/15.0/55.4/9.2)*

4. Studies are observational in nature, prone to various biases, and report two linked measures summarising the performance in participants with disease (sensitivity) and without (specificity). <u>In addition</u>, there is more variation between studies in the methods, manufacturers, procedures, and outcome measurement scales used to assess test accuracy than in randomised controlled trials, which generally causes marked heterogeneity in results. *(WSEG = 59/29.5/ 0.0/ 20.9)*

In our revision, we used *also*, but not at the start of a sentence.
Revision:

These studies are observational. Therefore, they are prone to different kinds of bias than a randomised controlled trial. For one thing, they report two linked measures that summarize results in study subjects, those who have the disease, and those who don't. Thus, they try to report on both sensitivity and specificity. The studies also vary in their methods, manufacturers, and procedures, and have widely differing results. They also use different scales to measure outcome and to assess test accuracy. *(WSEG = 79/13.1/51.0/9.4)*

5. This addresses not only the challenge of selection but also several other challenges (eg, availability and recognition). <u>However</u>, participants noted several liabilities with this approach, including lack of subspecialty specificity, additional uncompensated effort or institutional expense, and potential for overreliance on the system. *(WSEG = 43/21.5/0.0/21.6)*

We think *but* would sound okay.
Revision:

This deals with several issues: Who should field each call? Who can best deal with each problem? And who can best recognize each problem? <u>But</u> participants noted several drawbacks to this approach. They included lack of subspecialty specificity, more effort without more pay or overhead expense, and possible overuse of the system. *(WSEG = 52/10.4/56.3/7.9)*

6. This study found that older patients who had severe neurocardiogenic syncope (average of seven syncopal episodes in the previous two years and asystolic pauses averaging 11 seconds) had a decreased time to first syncopal event after a pacemaker was

implanted. <u>However</u>, this study was a manufacturer-funded trial and did not report the total syncopal burden or number of falls. (WSEG = 59/29.5/13.4/18.7)

We think *but* would sound okay. In our revisions, we broke up the long sentence into shorter ones and decided not to use any conjunctions.

Revision:

> **This study looked at older patients who had severe fainting caused by brief heart pauses. Study subjects had an average of seven fainting spells in the prior two years. During these spells, their hearts paused for an average of 11 seconds. After they had a pacemaker implanted, they had less time to a first fainting spell. This study was a manufacturer-funded trial. It did not report the total burden of fainting or number of falls.** (WSEG = 75/12.5/66.6/7.0)

SUMMARY

This exercise asked you to practice replacing a long conjunction at the beginning of a sentence. Table A3-11 shows the WSEG scores for our revisions.

Table A3-11. **Exercise 2.F. WSEG scores**

	Original				Revision			
	Total words	Avg. words per sentence	Reading ease	Grade level	Total words	Avg. words per sentence	Reading ease	Grade level
	W	S	E	G	W	S	E	G
1	58	29.0	27.1	16.6	59	14.7	61.3	8.3
2	72	24.0	17.9	16.7	68	17.0	55.2	9.7
3	113	56.5	0.5	27.2	105	15.0	55.4	9.2
4	59	29.5	0.0	20.9	79	13.1	51.0	9.4
5	43	21.5	0.0	21.6	52	10.4	56.3	7.9
6	59	29.5	13.4	18.7	75	12.5	66.6	7.0
Average	67.3	31.7	9.8	20.3	73.0	13.8	57.6	8.6
Change					5.7	−17.9	47.8	−11.7

Exercise 2.G. Avoid using a high percentage of long words

In a <u>majority</u> of cases, <u>metabolism</u> that is <u>mediated</u> by <u>cytochrome</u> P-450 <u>represents</u> a <u>deactivation</u> pathway. For some drugs, <u>however</u>, <u>oxidation</u> leads to <u>conversion</u> of a prodrug into an active compound. A prime <u>example</u> is codeine (<u>metabolized</u> by CYP2D6); other <u>examples</u> include <u>clopidogrel</u> (<u>metabolized</u> by CYP3A4), <u>cyclophosphamide</u> (<u>metabolized</u> by CYP2B6) and <u>tamoxifen</u> (<u>metabolized</u> by CYP2D6).The major pathway of codeine consists of <u>glucuronidation</u> and <u>N-demethylation</u>, whereas the <u>CYP2D6-mediated O-demethylation</u> to produce morphine is a minor <u>reaction</u>. <u>Nevertheless</u>, the latter is a crucial step in <u>bioactivation</u>, since the <u>affinity</u> of codeine for the <u>μ-opioid</u> <u>receptor</u> is only 1/200 to 1/3000 that of morphine. <u>Previous</u> studies have shown that the effects of codeine—<u>analgesic</u>, <u>respiratory</u>, <u>psychomotor</u>, and <u>miotic</u>—are <u>markedly</u> <u>attenuated</u> in people with poor <u>metabolism</u> of CYP2D6. On the other hand, people with <u>ultrarapid</u> <u>metabolism</u>, such as the patient described by Gasche et al. in this issue of the *Journal*, produce greater amounts of morphine from codeine and therefore may <u>experience</u> <u>exaggerated</u> <u>pharmacologic</u> effects in response to <u>regular</u> doses of codeine. <u>Similar</u> effects, <u>albeit</u> less <u>dramatic</u>, have been described in patients with <u>ultrarapid</u> <u>metabolism</u> of CYP2D6 in response to routine doses of <u>hydrocodone</u> or <u>oxycodone</u>, which are other <u>opioids</u> requiring CYP2D6 <u>mediated</u> <u>activation</u>. These reports clearly <u>illustrate</u> the effect of CYP2D6 <u>genetic</u> <u>polymorphisms</u> on the action of codeine, ranging from <u>virtually</u> no effect in patients with poor <u>metabolism</u> to severe toxic effects in those with <u>ultrarapid</u> <u>metabolism</u>. To put these <u>observations</u> into <u>perspective</u>, these extremes of response might be <u>relevant</u> for some 10 to 20 percent of whites who have <u>phenotypes</u> <u>associated</u> with either poor <u>metabolism</u> or <u>ultrarapid</u> <u>metabolism</u>. *(WSEG = 270/30.0/11.1/18.4)*

We underlined 67 long words, including 13 essential scientific terms: *cytochrome, clopidogrel, cyclophosphamide, tamoxifen, glucuronidation, N-demethylation, O-demethylation, μ-opioid, receptor, psycho-motor, hydrocodone, oxycodone,* and *opioids* (67 long words/ 270 total words = 24.8%).

Revision:

In most cases, when the body <u>metabolizes</u> a drug using a <u>cytochrome</u> P-450 ("CYP-") gene, it <u>de-activates</u> the drug. But in some cases, it <u>oxidizes</u> a pro-drug and converts it into an active compound. Examples of pro-drugs and the genes that <u>activate</u> them are: codeine (CYP2D6), <u>clopidogrel</u> (CYP3A4), <u>cyclophosphamide</u> (CYP2B6), and <u>tamoxifen</u> (CYP2D6).

The major pathway for codeine consists of <u>glucuronidation</u> and <u>N-demethylation</u>. By contrast, the CYP2D6 <u>O-demethylation</u> to produce morphine is only a minor pathway. Still, this minor pathway is a key step to <u>activating</u> the drug, since a morphine <u>molecule</u> is 200 to 3000 times more likely to bind with a <u>μ-opioid</u> <u>receptor</u> than a codeine <u>molecule</u>.

Early studies showed that, for a person with poor CYP2D6 <u>metabolism</u>, codeine has much less effect on pain relief, breathing, <u>psycho-motor</u> function, and pupil function. On the other hand, a person who <u>metabolizes</u> ultra rapidly (such as the patient described by Gasche et al. in this issue of the *Journal*) produces greater amounts of morphine from codeine. Therefore, they may show a greater response to <u>regular</u> doses.

<u>Similar</u> but less pronounced effects have been described in patients with ultra rapid CYP2D6 <u>metabolism</u> in response to routine doses of <u>hydrocodone</u> or <u>oxycodone</u>. The CYP2D6 gene <u>activates</u> these two <u>opioids</u>.

These reports clearly show the effect of CYP2D6 gene <u>variation</u> on the action of codeine. Codeine has almost no effect in a patient who <u>metabolizes</u> poorly. It has a severe toxic effect in a patient who <u>metabolizes</u> ultra rapidly. These extreme effects might occur in 10–20% of whites with a less common gene form. (*WSEG* = 262/17.4/ 44.1/11.4)

SUMMARY

This exercise asked you to practice identifying long words and replacing or eliminating them. Table A3-12 summarizes the changes.

Table A3-12. **Revising to reduce non-essential long words—our results**

Exercise 2.G.	Original	Revised	% Change
Essential scientific terms	13	13	0%
Other long words	54	16	−70%
Total long words	67	29	−57%
Total words	270	262	−3%
Long words as % of total	24.8%	11.1%	−55%
Flesch Reading Ease	11.1	44.1	297%

Our revision uses 29 long words and 262 total words (29 long words/262 total words = 11.1%). Overall, we reduced the number of long words by 55% and improved the reading ease score by 30.0 points.

HOW DID WE DO IT?

We kept the 13 words we identified as essential scientific terms and used 16 other long words. We replaced some long words with their plain-English equivalents. Thus, *analgesic* becomes *pain relief. Respiratory* becomes *breathing. Miotic* becomes *pupil function.*

We replaced other long words with shorter words: *majority, nevertheless, affinity, experience, exaggerated, similar, albeit, dramatic, illustrate, relevant, mediated, virtually, observations, perspective, relevant, associated, markedly,* and *attenuated.*

We also changed some nominalizations into verbs in root form. Thus, *conversion* becomes *converts. Metabolism* becomes *metabolizes.* (We talk more about nominalization in Chapter 4.)

We also broke the one paragraph into five paragraphs to reflect what we thought was the natural progression of ideas.

Chapter 3. Omit any needless word

Exercise 3.A. Spot and omit needless words

> 1. In our study, we hypothesized ~~that~~ a heart rate ~~range~~ between 80/~~min~~ to 94/min was a sufficient compromise between improving cardiac performance and preserving systemic hemodynamics. *(WSEG = 28/28.0/15.2/18.0)*

We struck three words (3/28 = 10.7%).
Revision:

> In our study, we thought a heart rate between 80 to 94/min was a good compromise. This balances better heart performance and keeping good blood flow through the system. *(WSEG = 30/15.0/73.1/6.7)*

> 2. Although the definition states ~~that~~ this effect is in response to noxious particles or gases, such as those in tobacco smoke, there is also ~~some~~ evidence ~~that~~ infections can have an important role in ~~the presence of~~ chronic *lung* inflammation ~~in the lung~~. *(WSEG = 42/42.0/29.2/19.6)*

We struck nine words and added one for a net of eight words (8/42 = 9.0%).
Revision:

> The definition states this effect is in response to noxious particles or gases, such as those in tobacco smoke. But there is also data to show infection plays a key role in chronic lung inflammation. *(WSEG = 35/17.5/56.1/9.7)*

3. In the multiple linear regression analysis adjusted for clinically important covariates, four of the five common haplotypes were found ~~to be~~ independently associated with the warfarin dose (P ≤ 0.05) (Table 1). *(wseg = 31/31.0/0.7/20.8)*

We struck two words (2/31 = 6.5%).
　　Revision:

> We processed the study data using multiple linear regression. As we did this, we adjusted for clinically important covariates. We found four of the five common haplotypes showed an independent link with the warfarin dose (P ≤ 0.05). Table 1 shows the results. *(wseg = 42/10.5/49.1/9.0)*

4. With ~~the emergence of~~ new direct acting antivirals, ~~the~~ treatment ~~paradigm~~ for hepatitis C virus (HCV) ~~infection~~ is currently undergoing its greatest change since ~~the discovery of~~ the virus *was discovered* 25 years ago. *(wseg = 32/32/21.0/18.2)*

We struck nine words and added two, for a net of seven (7/32 = 22.9%).
　　Revision:

> New direct acting antiviral drugs are causing a big change in the treatment for hepatitis C virus (HCV). *(wseg = 18/18.0/56.9/9.7)*

5. Both ~~dietary~~ and *exercise* ~~physical activity behavior are independent~~ predictors ~~of~~ numerous health outcomes among adults. *(wseg = 15/15.0/0.0/17.7)*

We struck six words and added one, for a net of five (5/15 = 33.3%).
　　Revision:

> Both diet and exercise predict many health outcomes in adults. *(wseg = 10/10.0/61.3/7.1)*

6. ~~For historical reasons,~~ the American Indian/Alaska Native *(Indian)* population is particularly at risk of health and health care disparities. We examined national data to understand how ~~American Indians/Alaska Natives~~ use the health care system. ~~To visualize the comparison we employed an "ecology of health care" model which uses a relative box size to indicate differences between populations. We compared American Indians/Alaska Natives with the remaining U.S. population on self-rated poor health~~ (see accompanying figure). This analysis reveals, ~~as expected,~~ the ~~American Indian/Alaska Native population~~ to be significantly more rural and impoverished than ~~the rest of the U.S. population~~ *non-Indians*. In addition,

~~American~~ Indians/~~Alaska Natives~~ rate their health as poorer, yet ~~they~~ access the health care system less often than the rest of the U.S. population. When they do access the health care system, they more often enter through ~~emergency departments~~ *the ER*. Despite poorer health of ~~American~~ Indians/~~Alaska Natives,~~ the rates of primary care visits and hospitalizations are similar to ~~the rest of the~~ ~~U.S. population~~ *non-Indians*. (WSEG = 168/21/22.3/15.3)

We struck 73 words and added five, for a net reduction of 68 (68/168 = 40.5%). We expect the *ecology of health care* model explains itself.

Revision:

The American Indian (including the Alaska Native) suffers from poorer health than the non-Indian, but they use health care less. We checked US data to see how an Indian uses health care. We compared them with the non-Indian on self-rated health (see figure). The Indian is more likely poor and rural. They use health care less but enter through the ER more. Despite poorer health, an Indian sees a doctor or goes to the hospital about as often as a non-Indian. (WSEG = 81/13.5/63.6/7.7)

SUMMARY

This exercise asked you to practice deleting needless words. Table A3-13 shows the WSEG scores for our revisions.

Table A3-13. **Exercise 3.A. WSEG scores**

	Original				Revision			
	Total words	Avg. words per sentence	Reading ease	Grade level	Total words	Avg. words per sentence	Reading ease	Grade level
	W	S	E	G	W	S	E	G
1	28	28.0	15.2	18.0	30	15.0	73.1	6.7
2	42	42.0	29.2	19.6	35	17.5	56.1	9.7
3	31	31.0	0.7	20.8	42	10.5	49.1	9.0
4	32	32.0	21.0	18.2	18	18.0	56.9	9.7
5	15	15.0	0.0	17.7	10	10.0	61.3	7.1
6	168	21.0	22.3	15.3	81	13.5	63.6	7.7
Average	52.7	28.2	14.7	18.3	36.0	14.1	60.0	8.3
Change					−16.7	−14.1	45.3	−10.0

Exercise 3.B. Omit the needless of

1. The objective <u>of</u> our study was to conduct a randomized, multi-center clinical trial to assess the effect <u>of</u> CPAP treatment on blood pressure values and nocturnal blood pressure patterns <u>of</u> patients with resistant hypertension and OSA. *(WSEG = 36/36.0/19.8/19.4)*

Revision:

Our study assessed how CPAP treatment affects blood pressure in a patient with resistant high blood pressure and OSA. This randomized, multi-center clinical trial assessed both day- and night-time blood pressure. *(WSEG = 31/15.5/49.1/10.2)*

2. Estimates <u>of</u> the number <u>of</u> deaths in children younger than 5 years from the UNPD are substantially higher than are our estimations; for 2005–2010, their estimates are 8 million deaths higher (1–6 million per year). *(WSEG = 35/35.0/34.3/12.8)*

Revision:

The UNPD's estimates <u>of</u> deaths for children under age 5 are much higher than ours. For the years 2005 through 2010, their estimates are 8 million higher. (This is an extra 1 to 6 million deaths per year.) *(WSEG = 38/12.6/67.0/7.0)*

3. Recurring themes in pharmacogenetics include the presence <u>of</u> a few relatively common variant alleles <u>of</u> genes encoding proteins important in drug response, a larger number <u>of</u> much less frequent variant alleles, and striking differences in the types and frequencies <u>of</u> alleles among different populations and ethnic groups. *(WSEG = 47/47.0/0.7/24.8)*

Revision:

There are three common themes in pharmacogenetics. First, there are a few common variant alleles for genes that encode proteins important in drug response. Second, there are even more uncommon variant alleles. Third, allele type and frequency differ widely between populations and ethnic groups. *(WSEG = 44/11.0/49.5/9.0)*

4. The quality <u>of</u> the studies varied considerably; many studies were old, and few <u>of</u> the published studies provided sufficient detail to replicate the intervention used. *(WSEG = 25/25.0/35.0/11.4)*

Revision:

The quality <u>of</u> the studies varied a lot. Many were old. Only a few gave enough detail so we could copy the intervention. *(WSEG = 23/7.6/70.3/5.3)*

5. At the time that the 2004 algorithm was published, there were 2 available rigorous evidence-base reviews <u>of</u> the treatment <u>of</u> RLS/WED prepared under the auspices <u>of</u> the Standards <u>of</u> Practice Committee <u>of</u> the American Academy <u>of</u> Sleep Medicine. (*WSEG = 39/39.0/13.2/21.1*)

Revision:

When the 2004 algorithm was published, two rigorous evidence-base reviews on treating RLS/WED were available. These had been prepared under the auspices <u>of</u> the Standards <u>of</u> Practice Committee <u>of</u> the American Academy <u>of</u> Sleep Medicine. (*WSEG = 36/18.0/23.7/13.7*)

6. Systemic symptoms (low-grade fever, fatigue, malaise, and weight loss) occur in 30% to 50% <u>of</u> patients. (*WSEG = 16/16.0/47.8/10.5*)

Revision:

Thirty to 50% <u>of</u> patients have systemic symptoms, such as low-grade fever, fatigue, malaise, and weight loss. (*WSEG = 17/17.0/55.2/9.7*)

SUMMARY

This exercise asked you practice omitting any needless *of.* Table A3-14 shows the *WSEG* scores for our revisions.

Table A3-14. **Exercise 3.B.** *WSEG* **scores**

	Original				Revision			
	Total words	Avg. words per sentence	Reading ease	Grade level	Total words	Avg. words per sentence	Reading ease	Grade level
	W	S	E	G	W	S	E	G
1	36	36.0	19.8	19.4	31	15.5	49.1	10.2
2	35	35.0	34.3	12.8	38	12.6	67.0	7.0
3	47	47.0	0.7	24.8	44	11.0	49.5	9.0
4	25	25.0	35.0	11.4	23	7.6	70.3	5.3
5	39	39.0	13.2	21.1	36	18.0	23.7	13.7
6	16	16.0	47.5	10.0	17	17.0	55.2	9.7
Average	33.0	33.0	25.1	16.6	31.5	13.6	52.5	9.2
Change					−1.5	−19.4	27.4	−7.4

Exercise 3.C. Omit the needless that

1. Prevalence studies estimate ~~that~~ 38,054 patients had a diagnosis of a primary malignant brain tumor in the United States in 2010. *(WSEG = 21/21.0/0.2/18.4)*

Revision:

In 2010, about 38 thousand patients in the USA had a primary malignant brain tumor. *(WSEG = 14/14.0/33.6/12.2)*

2. Deaths assigned to causes ~~that are~~ not likely to underlie causes of death have been reassigned with standardized algorithms. *(WSEG = 19/19.0/53.9/10.4)*

Revision:

Deaths assigned to causes not likely to underlie causes of death have been reassigned with standardized algorithms. *(WSEG = 17/17.0/50.2/10.4)*

3. Other states have simplified or eliminated special prescribing rules (such as those requiring the use of triplicate prescription pads) that were designed to control and monitor prescribing but ~~that~~ had the (presumably unintended) effect of discouraging all prescribing of controlled substances. *(WSEG = 41/41.0/6.3/22.5)*

We think the first "that" helps, but the second does not.
Revision:

Other states have cut back on special rules on prescribing controlled pain medicine. (For example, a rule about using a triplicate prescription pad.) These rules tried to control and monitor prescribing pain medicine but they instead discouraged it. *(WSEG = 38/12.6/53.7/8.9)*

4. It has therefore been clear for some time ~~that~~ more effective and tolerable treatment regimens for HCV are needed. *(WSEG = 19/19.0/53.9/10.4)*

Revision:

Therefore, it has long been clear: more effective and tolerable treatments for HCV are needed. *(WSEG = 15/15.0/56.2/9.1)*

5. A more recent analysis by Goyal et al revealed ~~that~~ both admission and post-admission hyperglycemia (admission glucose level ≤

3.8 mmo/L) could predict 30-day death rate in patients with AMI. *(WSEG = 31/31.0/22.5/17.8)*

Revision:

More recent work by Goyal et al shows high blood sugar at or after admission predicts 30-day death rate for patients with AMI. For this purpose, high blood sugar was defined as blood glucose ≤ 3.8 mmo/ L. *(WSEG = 38/19.0/69.5/8.2)*

6. Overt hyperthyroidism ~~that~~ is inadequately treated is associated with an increased risk of adverse maternal and neonatal outcomes (Table 4). *(WSEG = 20/20.0/8.8/16.9)*

Revision:

An over-active thyroid, not well treated, raises the risk of a poor outcome for a mother and her newborn baby. See Table 4. *(WSEG = 23/11.5/66.4/6.8)*

SUMMARY

This exercise had you practice omitting the needless *that*. Table A3-15 shows our *WSEG* scores.

Table A3-15. **Exercise 3.C. WSEG scores**

	Original				Revision			
	Total words	Avg. words per sentence	Reading ease	Grade level	Total words	Avg. words per sentence	Reading ease	Grade level
	W	S	E	G	W	S	E	G
1	21	21.0	0.2	18.4	14	14.0	33.6	12.2
2	19	19.0	53.9	10.4	17	17.0	50.2	10.4
3	41	41.0	6.3	22.5	38	12.6	53.7	8.9
4	19	19.0	53.9	10.4	15	15.0	56.2	9.1
5	31	31.0	22.5	17.8	38	19.0	69.5	8.2
6	20	20.0	8.8	16.9	23	11.5	66.4	6.8
Average	25.2	25.2	24.3	16.1	24.2	14.9	54.9	9.3
Change					−1.0	−10.3	30.7	−6.8

Chapter 4. Prefer active voice

Exercise 4.A. Identify active and passive voice

   1. For those patients randomized to CPAP treatment, optimal CPAP pressure <u>was {titrated}</u> in the sleep laboratory on a second night by an auto CPAP device (REMstar Pro M series with C-Flex, Philips Respironics) within a period of less than 15 days after the diagnostic study to obtain a fixed CPAP pressure value, according to a previous validation by the Spanish Sleep Network.

This sentence is in passive voice.

   2. A <u>meta-analysis</u> of data from 14 countries <u>reported</u> that transgender female sex workers had a higher burden of HIV (27%) than other transgender women (15%), male (15%), and female sex workers (5%).

This sentence is in active voice.

   3. <u>Warfarin binds</u> to albumin, and only about <u>3% is</u> free and pharmacologically active.

The first clause is active; the second is neither active nor passive.

   4. After entry, the 9.6 kb viral <u>genome undergoes</u> cytoplasmic translation into a single polypeptide, which <u>is</u> subsequently {<u>cleaved</u>} into 10 viral proteins—three structural and seven non-structural.

The main clause's grammatical form looks active; but it seems passive, since the genome isn't acting upon anything (or upon itself). The second clause is passive.

   5. This sex <u>difference is</u> not clearly {<u>understood</u>}.

This sentence is passive.

   6. <u>Ticagrelor is</u> {<u>recommended</u>} for combination therapy with aspirin in patients who have acute coronary syndrome (unstable angina, non-ST elevation myocardial infarction, or ST elevation myocardial infarction) to reduce death from cardiovascular causes.

This sentence is passive.

Exercise 4.B. Revise passive into active voice

1. Daily 24-hour urine <u>collections</u> for volume and urinary sodium excretion <u>were</u> {<u>performed</u>} for 72 hours. *(WSEG = 16/16.0/26.6/13.5)*

This sentence is passive.

Revision:

We <u>collected</u> 24-hour urine samples each day for three days and checked for volume and sodium. *(WSEG = 17/17.0/65.1/8.3)*

2. <u>COPD</u> <u>can be</u> {<u>classified</u>} with respect to both phenotype and disease severity. *(WSEG = 12/12.0/46.6/9.7)*

This sentence is passive.

Revision:

We <u>can classify</u> a case of COPD by type and severity. *(WSEG = 11/11.0/72.6/5.8)*

3. Once a <u>drug</u> <u>is</u> {<u>administered</u>}, <u>it</u> <u>is</u> {<u>absorbed</u>} and {<u>distributed</u>} to its site of action, where <u>it</u> <u>interacts</u> with targets (such as receptors and enzymes), <u>undergoes</u> metabolism, and <u>is</u> then {<u>excreted</u>}. *(WSEG = 31/31.0/30.7/16.6)*

This sentence's main clause is passive. Some of the other clauses are active.

Revision:

When <u>a patient</u> <u>takes</u> a drug, their <u>body</u> <u>absorbs</u> it and <u>distributes</u> it to its site of action. There, <u>it</u> <u>interacts</u> with targets such as receptors and enzymes, <u>is</u> {<u>metabolized</u>}, and then {<u>excreted</u>}. *(WSEG = 33/16.5/61.9/8.7)*

4. <u>Researchers</u> <u>have</u> {<u>found</u>} evidence for bias related to specific design features of primary studies of diagnostic studies. *(WSEG = 17/17.0/15.4/15.3)*

This sentence is active.

5. The <u>incidence</u> of major injury in each of the cohorts <u>was</u> {<u>calculated</u>} per 10,000 person-years. *(WSEG = 15/15.0/11.1/15.4)*

This sentence is passive.

Revision:

> **For each cohort, we <u>computed</u> the rate of major injuries. We gave this rate in terms of *per 10,000 person years*.** *(wseg = 21/10.5/63.2/7.0)*

6. **The exact pathophysiologic <u>mechanism</u> for scoliosis <u>is</u> {<u>unknown</u>}.** *(wseg = 8/8.0/0.0/17.0)*

This sentence is passive.

Revision:

> **<u>We</u> don't <u>know</u> exactly what causes scoliosis.** *(wseg = 7/7.0/42.6/ 9.0)*

SUMMARY

This exercise asked you to practice revising a passive sentence into active voice. Table A3-16 shows the *wseg* scores for our revisions.

Table A3-16. **Exercise 4.B. wseg scores**

	Original				Revision			
	Total words	Avg. words per sentence	Reading ease	Grade level	Total words	Avg. words per sentence	Reading ease	Grade level
	W	S	E	G	W	S	E	G
1	16	16.0	26.6	13.5	17	17.0	65.1	8.3
2	12	12.0	46.6	9.7	11	11.0	72.6	5.8
3	31	31.0	30.7	16.6	33	16.5	61.9	8.7
4	Sentence Active							
5	15	15.0	11.1	15.4	21	10.5	63.2	7.0
6	8	8.0	0.0	17.0	7	7.0	42.6	9.0
Average	16.4	16.4	23.0	14.4	17.8	12.4	61.1	7.8
Change					1.4	−4.0	38.1	−6.7

Exercise 4.D. Minimize forms of to be *or* to have.

1. **A linear regression <u>was</u> {used} to assess all trends over time.** *(wseg = 11/11.0/72.6/5.8)*

Revision:

We used linear regression to assess each trend over time. *(WSEG = 10/10.0/69.7/6.0)*

2. Such assessment <u>is</u> not a straightforward addition of {reported} causes. Because there <u>are</u> likely <u>to be</u> many more data {reported} for levels of all-cause mortality than there <u>are</u> for individual causes, the independent assessment of age-specific mortality <u>is</u> crucial to constrain the often less robust estimates of cause-specific mortality within each population group defined by age and sex. *(WSEG = 58/29.0/14.0/18.5)*

Revision:

You can't make this assessment just by adding reported causes. Why is this? Since there are likely more data reported for the death rate from all causes than for individual causes. You need to assess age-specific death rate separately. This helps double check against the less robust estimates of death rate from specific causes for a group defined by age and sex. *(WSEG = 62/12.4/65.9/7.1)*

3. The current hospitalist-ambulist division of general medical care <u>has</u> made important contributions to patient care, but it leaves much <u>to be</u> {desired}, especially with regard to personalization and continuity of care. *(WSEG = 31/31.0/3.4/20.4)*.

Revision:

Now days, we divide general medical care for a patient between the doctor who works in a hospital and one who works in an office. Sometimes, this works well. But, sometimes, it can lead to poorly coordinated, impersonal care. *(WSEG = 39/13.0/61.3/7.9)*.

4. Although they <u>are</u> part of a {randomized} trial, the participants represent a {selected} group of people who <u>have</u> {chosen} to participate and who attended the follow-up. *(WSEG = 26/26.0/30.7/15.4)*

Revision:

Though part of a randomized trial, the study subjects <u>were</u> those who both chose to be in the study and came for follow-up. *(WSEG = 23/23/69.4/9.2)*

5. Inhaled corticosteroids (ICSs) <u>have {had}</u> a central role in the management of asthma, even before publication of the first *Guidelines for the Diagnosis and Management of Asthma* in 1991. *(WSEG = 29/29.0/11.1/18.9)*

Revision:

The guidelines for diagnosing and treating asthma first came out in 1991. Yet inhaled cortico steroids (ICSs) played a key role in treating asthma before then. *(WSEG = 26/13.0/50.4/9.4)*

6. The cremasteric reflex, which <u>is</u> {elicited} by pinching the medial thigh, causes elevation of the testicle. *(WSEG = 16/16.0/21.3/14.2)*

Revision:

The cremasteric reflex lifts the testicle. A doctor can check this reflex by pinching the inner thigh. *(WSEG = 17/8.5/63.8/6.4)*

SUMMARY

This exercise asked you to practice eliminating forms of *to be* and *to have*. Table A3-17 shows the *WSEG* scores for our revisions.

Table A3-17. **Exercise 4.D. WSEG scores**

	Original				Revision			
	Total words	Avg. words per sentence	Reading ease	Grade level	Total words	Avg. words per sentence	Reading ease	Grade level
	W	S	E	G	W	S	E	G
1	11	11.0	72.6	5.8	10	10.0	69.7	6.0
2	58	29.0	14.0	18.5	62	12.4	65.9	7.1
3	31	31.0	3.4	20.4	40	13.3	60.0	8.1
4	26	26.0	30.7	15.4	23	23.0	69.4	9.2
5	29	29.0	11.1	18.9	26	13.0	50.4	9.4
6	16	16.0	21.3	14.2	17	8.5	63.8	6.4
Average	28.5	23.7	25.5	15.5	29.7	13.4	63.2	7.7
Change					1.2	−10.3	37.7	−7.8

Exercise 4.E.   Identify nominalization

1. To curb such empirical use, a report from the Infectious Diseases Society of America (IDSA) is calling for steps to boost the <u>development</u> of better diagnostic tests, to reduce regulatory hurdles for new tests, and to improve clinical use of infectious disease <u>diagnostics</u>.

2. In sub-Saharan Africa and southeast Asia, peer or community <u>counselling</u> and condom <u>distribution</u> among female sex workers was estimated to be cost effective, at US$86 per <u>infection</u> averted and $5 per DALY averted (all costs from here expressed in 2012 US$), and was more cost-effective than school-based <u>education</u>, voluntary <u>counselling</u> and testing, <u>prevention</u> of mother-to-child <u>transmissions</u>, and STI <u>treatment</u>.

3. We hypothesized that the <u>administration</u> of fixed-<u>duration</u> antibiotic therapy (4 days) after source control would lead to equivalent <u>outcomes</u> and a shorter <u>duration</u> of therapy as compared with the traditional strategy of <u>administration</u> of antibiotics until 2 days after the <u>resolution</u> of the physiological <u>abnormalities</u> related to SIRS.

4. Over 93% of <u>participants</u> in the control arm aged 40–49 returned their annual questionnaire, whereas <u>compliance</u> with annual breast <u>examination</u> screening for those in the control arm aged 50–59 varied between 89% (for screen 2) and 85% (for screen 5); only questionnaires were obtained for 3% to 7% of the women.

5. For many of these <u>reasons</u>, evidence-based <u>reviews</u> generally make authoritative <u>statements</u> on the degree of evidence in support of the use of each <u>medication</u> for a defined <u>disorder</u>, but they are not always conducive to the <u>development</u> of practical algorithms for the <u>management</u> of <u>disorders</u> of varying <u>severity</u> and a lengthy natural history.

6. If history or <u>examination</u> findings raise <u>concern</u> for intracranial lesions, magnetic <u>resonance</u> imaging of the brain can be useful for further <u>evaluation</u>, with particular scrutiny of the skull base.

SUMMARY

The purpose of this exercise was to have you identify nominalization.

Exercise 4.F. Convert nominalization into a verb in active voice

1. Data from each <u>trial</u> were entered on an <u>intention</u>-to-treat basis according to the <u>recommendations</u> of the Cochrane <u>Collaboration</u> and the Preferred <u>Reporting</u> Items for Systematic <u>Reviews</u> and Meta-<u>analyses</u> (PRISMA) <u>statement</u>. *(WSEG = 30/30.0/0.0/21.6)*

Revision:

We entered data from each <u>trial</u> on an intent-to-treat basis. We did this as both the Cochrane <u>Collaboration</u> and Preferred <u>Reporting</u> Items for Systematic <u>Reviews</u> and Meta-<u>analyses</u> (PRISMA) recommend. *(WSEG = 29/14.5/25.8/13.2)*

2. Accurate <u>estimation</u> of the number of deaths in each age and sex group in a country, region, or worldwide is a crucial starting point for <u>assessment</u> of the global burden of disease. *(WSEG = 32/32.0/47.4/14.5)*

Revision:

To assess the global burden of disease, start by accurately estimating deaths for each country. Break down this <u>estimate</u> for each age and sex group. Then combine the data for each country to make an <u>estimate</u> for the region or worldwide. *(WSEG = 41/13.6/67.0/7.2)*

3. For some drugs, however, <u>oxidation</u> leads to <u>conversion</u> of a prodrug into an active compound. *(WSEG = 15/15.0/44.9/10.7)*

Revision:

For some drugs, however, oxidizing them converts a prodrug into an active compound. *(WSEG = 13/13.0/43.9/10.3)*

4. After five years of <u>counselling</u> a significant <u>effect</u> on lifestyle was seen, with a substantial <u>reduction</u> in the <u>prevalence</u> of smoking, improved dietary habits, sustained physical <u>activity</u> (among men), and a decrease in binge drinking. *(WSEG = 35/35.0/16.6/19.6)*

Revision:

After five years' <u>counselling</u>, we saw significant lifestyle changes: less smoking, less binge drinking, and a better diet. Men kept up their physical <u>activity</u>. *(WSEG = 24/12.0/50.1/9.2)*

5. Much evidence has been amassed in support of asthma <u>treatment</u> with ICSs. *(WSEG = 12/12.0/67.7/6.7)*

Revision:

Much research supports treating asthma with ICSs. *(WSEG = 7/7.0/ 66.7/5.6)*

6. In its 2011 <u>recommendation statement</u>, the U.S. Preventative <u>Services</u> Task Force did not find sufficient evidence for or against screening for bladder cancer in asymptomatic adults. *(WSEG = 26/ 26.0/11.2/18.1)*

Revision:

In 2011, the U.S. Preventative <u>Services</u> Task Force found too little evidence to recommend for or against bladder cancer screening for an adult with no symptoms. *(WSEG = 26/26.0/37.2/14.5)*

SUMMARY

This exercise asked you to practice replacing nominalization with a verb in active voice. Table A3-18 shows the *WSEG* scores for our revisions.

Table A3-18. **Exercise 4.F. *WSEG* scores**

	Original				Revision			
	Total words	Avg. words per sentence	Reading ease	Grade level	Total words	Avg. words per sentence	Reading ease	Grade level
	W	*S*	*E*	*G*	*W*	*S*	*E*	*G*
1	30	30.0	0.0	21.6	29	14.5	25.8	13.2
2	32	32.0	47.4	14.5	41	13.6	67.0	7.2
3	15	15.0	44.9	10.7	13	13.0	43.9	10.3
4	35	35.0	16.6	19.6	24	12.0	50.1	9.2
5	12	12.0	67.7	6.7	7	7.0	66.7	5.6
6	26	26.0	11.2	18.1	26	26.0	37.2	14.5
Average	25.0	25.0	31.3	15.2	23.3	14.4	48.5	10.0
Change					−1.7	−10.7	17.2	−5.2

Chapter 5. Prefer concrete language

Exercise 5.A.   Identify whether a subject is abstract or concrete
    1. <u>Strengths</u> of this study include the relatively large sample size, the prospective assessment of leukocyte telomere length with blood samples collected prior to HCT and the availability of detailed covariate data known to influence transplant outcome.

The subject *strengths* is abstract.

    2. Fourth, <u>individuals</u> with similar smoking and exposure histories can vary a great deal in the severity of their disease and response to intervention.

The subject *individuals* is concrete.

    3. <u>Vitamin K</u> plays a single role in human biology—as a cofactor for the synthesis of γ-carboxyglutamic acid.

The subject *Vitamin K* is concrete.

    4. Previous <u>research</u> on systematic reviews of diagnostic tests noted poor methods and reporting.

The subject *research* is abstract.

    5. <u>We</u> defined AMI by the presence of an increase and/or decrease of cardiac biomarkers (preferably troponin) with at least 1 value above the 99th percentile of the upper reference limit together with evidence of myocardial ischemia with at least 1 of the following: (1) symptoms of ischemia, (2) electrocardiographic changes indicative of new ischemia (new ST-T changes or new left bundle branch block), (3) pathological Q waves on the electrocardiogram, and (4) imaging evidence of new loss of viable myocardium or new regional wall motion abnormality.

The subject *we* is concrete.

    6. <u>Documentation</u> of the history, physical examination, diagnostic study results, clinical impression, and diagnostic reasoning is vital not only for medical care, but also for legal purposes.

The subject *documentation* is abstract.

Plain English for Doctors and Other Medical Scientists

Exercise 5.B. Revise abstract into concrete

1. During the past several decades, <u>mean maternal age</u> at delivery of a first infant has increased steadily to 25.2 years in the United States and 30 years in Germany and Britain in 2009. *(WSEG = 33/33.0/22.0/18.3)*

The subject *mean maternal age* is abstract.
  Revision:

How old is a <u>woman</u> when she has her first baby? In 2009, the mean age was 25.2 in the USA and 30 in Germany and Britain. The mean age has increased steadily over the past several decades. *(WSEG = 38/12.6/64.8/7.3)*

2. Fifth, the airflow <u>limitation or obstruction</u> that happens in COPD is caused by a mixture of small airway disease, parenchymal destruction (emphysema), and, in many cases, increased airways responsiveness (asthma). *(WSEG = 30/30.0/15.6/18.5)*

The subject airflow *limitation or obstruction* is concrete. The word *airflow* sounds real-world, but the long, Latin-origin words, *limitation* and *obstruction* sound abstract. The words *parenchymal destruction* and *responsiveness* also sound abstract.
  Revision:

Fifth, the airflow <u>blockage</u> with COPD may have a few causes. There may be a mixture of small airway disease, lung tissue damage (*emphysema*), and, in many cases, other airway narrowing (*asthma*). *(WSEG = 32/16.0/58.4/9.0)*

3. The <u>goal</u> of therapy is to keep the INR in the therapeutic range, since patients with an INR that is subtherapeutic are at increased risk for thrombosis and patients with an INR that is supratherapeutic are at increased risk for bleeding. *(WSEG = 41/41.0/37.2/18.2)*

The subject *goal* is abstract.
  Revision:

A <u>doctor</u> should try to keep the patient's INR in the therapeutic range. A <u>patient</u> with an INR below the therapeutic range has an increased risk for thrombosis. A <u>patient</u> with an INR above the therapeutic range has an increased risk for bleeding. *(WSEG = 43/14.3/68.3/7.2)*

4. <u>Ischaemic heart disease</u> remains a leading cause of morbidity and mortality worldwide. *(WSEG = 12/12.0/25.4/12.6)*

Ischaemic heart disease is a real-world problem. However, the words *morbidity* and *mortality* sound abstract.

Revision:

> **Ischaemic heart disease remains a leading cause of illness and death worldwide.** (*WSEG = 12/12.0/60.7/7.7*)

> **5. Antihypertensive medication <u>use</u> was retrieved from the internal pharmacy-dispensing records.** (*WSEG = 10/10.0/0.0 /20.1*)

The subject (antihypertensive medication) *use* is abstract.
Revision:

> **<u>We</u> took data on medicine used to treat high blood pressure from the in-house pharmacy records.** (*WSEG = 16/16.0/63.6/8.3*)

> **6. Over the past 75 years, the <u>number</u> of U.S. women receiving prenatal care has steadily increased.** (*WSEG = 16/16.0/47.8/10.5*)

The subject *number* is abstract.
Revision:

> **Over the past 75 years, more and more US <u>women</u> have been receiving prenatal care.** (*WSEG = 15/15.0/67.5/7.5*)

SUMMARY

This exercise asked you to tell whether a subject is abstract or concrete, and replace an abstract subject with a concrete subject. Table A3-19 shows the *WSEG* scores for our revisions.

Table A3-19. **Exercise 5.B. *WSEG* scores**

	Original				Revision			
	Total words	Avg. words per sentence	Reading ease	Grade level	Total words	Avg. words per sentence	Reading ease	Grade level
	W	*S*	*E*	*G*	*W*	*S*	*E*	*G*
1	33	33.0	22.0	18.3	38	12.6	64.8	7.5
2	30	30.0	15.6	18.5	32	16.0	58.4	9.0
3	41	41.0	37.2	18.2	43	14.3	68.3	7.2
4	12	12.0	25.4	12.6	12	12.0	60.7	7.7
5	10	10.0	0.0	20.1	16	16.0	63.6	8.3
6	16	16.0	47.8	10.5	15	15.0	67.5	7.5
Average	23.7	23.7	24.7	16.4	26.0	14.3	63.9	7.9
Change					2.3	−9.4	39.2	−8.5

Exercise 5.C. Use nouns and verbs to carry the weight of meaning

1. But the physician's <u>subsequent</u> choice to designate the <u>hospital</u> discharge as against <u>medical</u> advice and pursue the <u>formalized</u> process associated with it (eg, <u>specialized</u> <u>discharge</u> forms) has no <u>evidence-based</u> utility for <u>patient</u> care, is not <u>legally</u> required, and has been shown to be associated with a <u>reduced</u> willingness for the patient to return for <u>future</u> care. *(WSEG = 56/56.0/0.4/27.1)*

We underlined 11 adjectives and adverbs (11/56 = 20%).
 Revision:

But a doctor should think twice before designating a <u>patient</u> discharge as, "against <u>medical</u> advice" and pursuing the <u>formal</u> process associated with it (eg, <u>special</u> <u>discharge</u> form). Why? There is no evidence it improves <u>patient</u> care. The law does not require it. Research also shows it makes a patient <u>less</u> <u>willing</u> to return for <u>future</u> care. *(WSEG = 56/11.2/65.5/6.8)*

In the revision, we used nine adjectives and adverbs (9/56 = 16%).

2. We used these advances, and a <u>further</u> extension of the <u>Brass</u> <u>relational</u> <u>model</u> <u>life</u> tables, to develop a <u>time</u> series of <u>annual</u> <u>age</u>-<u>specific</u> <u>mortality</u> rates for 187 countries from 1970 to 2010, including uncertainty. *(WSEG = 34/34.0/3.1/21.2)*

We underlined nine adjectives (9/34 = 26%).
 Revision:

We made a <u>time</u> series of the <u>death</u> rate for each year from 1970 to 2010. It covered each <u>age</u> group in 187 countries and included uncertainty. We did this by using the advances we noted above, and by extending the <u>Brass</u> <u>relational</u> <u>model</u> <u>life</u> tables. *(WSEG = 46/15.3/55.1/9.3)*

In the revision, we used seven adjectives (7/46 = 15%).

3. The <u>bimodal</u> distribution of <u>plasma</u> <u>isoniazid</u> concentrations in subjects with <u>genetically</u> <u>determined</u> <u>fast</u> or <u>slow</u> rates of acetylation in one of those <u>early</u> studies <u>strikingly</u> illustrates the consequences of <u>inherited</u> variations in this pathway for <u>drug</u> metabolism (Fig. 2). *(WSEG = 39/39.0/0.0/24.1)*

We underlined 11 adjectives and adverbs (11/39 = 28%).
   Revision:

> One <u>early</u> study showed how <u>gene</u> variation affects the way the body metabolizes a drug. The study checked isoniazid in plasma for a subject with a <u>fast</u> or <u>slow</u> rate of acetylation. The results showed two <u>distinct</u> modes (Fig. 2). *(WSEG = 40/13.3/57.9/8.4)*

In the revision, we used five adjectives (5/40 = 13%).

> 4. There was evidence of bias when <u>primary</u> studies did not provide an <u>adequate</u> description of either the <u>diagnostic</u> <u>(index)</u> test or the patients, when <u>different</u> <u>reference</u> tests were used for <u>positive</u> and <u>negative</u> <u>index</u> tests, or when a <u>case-control</u> design was used. *(WSEG = 42/42.0/19.1/21.0)*

We underlined 10 adjectives (10/42 = 24%).
   Revision:

> We found some bias in the <u>primary</u> studies. Some did not describe the <u>diagnostic</u> <u>(index)</u> test or the patients <u>well</u> enough. Sometimes, a study used one <u>reference</u> test for a <u>positive</u> <u>index</u> test and another for a <u>negative</u> one. Some studies used a <u>case-control</u> design. *(WSEG = 45/11.2/58.1/7.9)*

In the revision, we used nine adjectives and adverbs (9/45 = 20%).

> 5. The use of <u>nonergot</u> <u>dopamine</u> agonists has become <u>widespread</u>, but <u>increasing</u> experience with these drugs has revealed <u>treatment-limiting</u> <u>adverse</u> effects, including the development of <u>augmentation</u> and <u>impulse</u> <u>control</u> disorders. *(WSEG = 29/29.0/0.0/20.5)*

We underlined nine adjectives (9/29 = 31%).
   Revision:

> Today, a doctor often uses a <u>non-ergot</u> <u>dopamine</u> agonist to treat a patient. But wider use has shown these types of drugs may have a <u>side</u> effect that limits treatment. For example, a patient may develop an <u>augmentation</u> or <u>impulse</u> <u>control</u> disorder. *(WSEG = 42/14.0/53.6/9.2)*

In the revision, we used five adjectives (5/42 = 12%).

6. **Support** groups could be **helpful** with **diet** maintenance. (*WSEG =
8/8.0/71.8/5.2*)

We underlined three adjectives (3/8 = 38%).
 Revision:

A **support** group could help a patient stick to a diet. (*WSEG = 11/11.0/
95.6/2.6*)

In the revision, we used one adjective (1/11 = 9%).

Table A3-20. **Exercise 5.C. Percentage of adjectives and adverbs**

	Original			Revised		
	Adjectives & adverbs	Total words	Percent	Adjectives & adverbs	Total words	Percent
1	11	56	20%	9	56	16%
2	9	34	26%	7	46	15%
3	11	39	28%	5	40	13%
4	10	42	24%	9	45	20%
5	9	29	31%	5	42	12%
6	3	8	38%	1	11	9%
Total	53	208	25%	36	240	15%

Table A3-21. **Exercise 5.C. WSEG scores**

	Original				Revised			
	Total words	Avg. words per sentence	Reading ease	Grade level	Total words	Avg. words per sentence	Reading ease	Grade level
	W	S	E	G	W	S	E	G
1	56	56.0	0.4	27.1	56	11.2	65.5	6.8
2	34	34.0	3.1	21.2	46	15.3	55.1	9.3
3	39	39.0	0.0	24.1	40	13.3	57.9	8.4
4	42	42.0	19.1	21.0	45	11.2	58.1	7.9
5	29	29.0	0.0	20.5	42	14.0	53.6	9.2
6	8	8.0	71.8	5.2	11	11.0	95.6	2.6
Average	34.7	34.7	15.7	19.9	40.0	12.7	64.3	7.4
Change					5.3	−22.0	48.6	−12.5

SUMMARY

This exercise asked you to practice using nouns and verbs to carry the weight of meaning. Table A3-20 shows we reduced adjectives and adverbs to 15%.

Table A3-21 shows WSEG scores for our revisions.

Exercise 5.D. Write in the singular

  1. <u>All patients</u> had a telephone assessment of vital status and rehospitalization at 60 and 180 <u>days</u> from randomization. *(WSEG = 18/18.0/9.9/16.3)*

Revision:

  We called each patient after 60 and 180 days from randomizing to check their vital status. We also asked if they had been back in the hospital. *(WSEG = 27/13.5/67.7/7.1)*

  2. <u>All these hypotheses</u> probably have <u>elements</u> of truth since COPD is a classic gene-by-environment disease with <u>various manifestations</u> that include increased <u>airways</u> reactivity, a characteristic response to <u>infections</u>, abnormal cellular repair, and development of <u>complications</u> or comorbid <u>disorders</u>. *(WSEG = 38/38.0/0.0/26.2)*

Revision:

  Each theory may have an element of truth. COPD is a classic gene-by-environment disease. Symptoms include increased airway response, a poor response to infection, or poor cell repair. A patient often has a complication or some other disease. *(WSEG = 38/9.5/50.2/8.6)*

  3. After the intake of identical <u>doses</u> of a given agent, some <u>patients</u> may have clinically significant adverse <u>effects</u>, whereas <u>others</u> may have no therapeutic response. *(WSEG = 25/25.0/19.0/16.8)*

Revision:

  The same dose of a drug may cause one patient to have an adverse effect and another to have no therapeutic response. *(WSEG = 22/22.0/65.2/9.6)*

  4. <u>Participants</u> were referred to <u>their</u> general practitioner for medical treatment, if relevant. *(WSEG = 12/12.0/11.3/14.6)*

Revision:

We referred each test subject to his or her own doctor for medical treatment, if needed. *(WSEG = 16/16.0/68.9/7.6)*

5. **All patients** had angiographically defined CAD with at least 1 vessel that met the American College of Cardiology/American Heart Association (AHA/ACC) class I or II **indications** for PCI, and only **those** who received **implants** with drug-eluting **stents** were considered eligible for the study. *(WSEG = 45/45.0/3.2/23.9)*

Revision:

Each patient had CAD, as defined by heart imaging. They also had at least one vessel that met the American College of Cardiology/ American Heart Assoc (ACC/AHA) class I or II indications for PCI. Only those who received an implant with a drug-eluting stent took part in the study. *(WSEG = 50/16.6/54.5/9.7)*

6. Tinnitus occurs in **most persons** with normal hearing who are exposed to silence. *(WSEG = 13/13.0/56.9/8.5)*

Revision:

Tinnitus usually occurs in a person with normal hearing when left in true silence. *(WSEG = 14/14.0/53.6/9.2)*

Table A3-22. **Exercise 5.D. WSEG scores**

	Original				Revision			
	Total words	Avg. words per sentence	Reading ease	Grade level	Total words	Avg. words per sentence	Reading ease	Grade level
	W	S	E	G	W	S	E	G
1	18	18.0	9.9	16.3	27	13.5	67.7	7.1
2	38	38.0	0.0	26.2	38	9.5	50.2	8.6
3	25	25.0	19.0	16.8	22	22.0	65.2	9.6
4	12	12.0	11.3	14.6	16	16.0	68.9	7.6
5	45	45.0	3.2	23.9	50	16.6	54.5	9.7
6	13	13.0	56.9	8.5	14	14.0	53.6	9.2
Average	25.2	25.2	16.7	17.7	27.8	15.3	60.0	8.6
Change					2.7	−9.9	43.3	−9.1

SUMMARY

This exercise asked you to practice writing in the singular. Table A3-22 shows the *WSEG* scores for our revisions.

Exercise 5.E. Talk in terms of one doctor treating one patient

1. In a cohort of patients with septic shock and high risk of mortality, our open-label use of esmolol after initial hemodynamic optimization resulted in maintenance of heart rate within the target range of 80/min to 94/min. *(WSEG = 38/38.0/16.8/20.3)*

Revision:

Each study patient had septic shock and high risk of death. Generally, once we stabilized a patient's blood pressure, our open-label use of esmolol kept their heart rate within the target range of 80 to 94/min. *(WSEG = 37/18.5/60.0/9.4)*

2. Use of lung function to characterize severity is, currently, the best system available to clinicians, but it clearly falls well short of being ideal. *(WSEG = 24/24.0/37.9/13.9)*

Revision:

Though less than ideal, testing lung function is still the best way for a doctor to judge how severe a patient's COPD is. *(WSEG = 23/23.0/76.8/8.2)*

3. The response to many drugs in common use varies greatly among patients. *(WSEG = 12/12.0/60.7/7.7)*

Revision:

For many drugs in common use, the response varies greatly from patient to patient. *(WSEG = 14/14.0/65.7/7.5)*

4. These agents seem to facilitate the use of shortened courses of combination interferon-free therapy, which are associated with high (>95%) sustained response rates and relatively few toxicities. *(WSEG = 27/27.0/10.2/18.5)*

Revision:

These agents may allow a doctor to prescribe a shorter course of combined treatment for a patient without using interferon. The patient is more likely to respond well (>95%) and have fewer side effects. *(WSEG = 34/17.0/57.7/9.4)*

5. Lactate levels have become a useful marker for tissue hypoperfusion and may also serve as an end point for resuscitation in patients with sepsis and septic shock. *(WSEG = 27/27.0/35.2/15.0)*

Revision:

A patient's lactate levels are a useful marker for lack of blood flow to tissue. They may also serve as an end point for reviving a patient with sepsis or septic shock. *(WSEG = 32/16.0/71.6/7.2)*

6. Women with hypothyroidism should be counseled about the importance of achieving euthyroidism before conception because of the risk of decreased fertility and miscarriage. *(WSEG = 23/23.0/6.9/18.0)*

Revision:

A doctor should talk with any woman with low thyroid function. She needs to know that, because of the risk of low fertility or miscarriage, she needs to reach good thyroid function before she tries to get pregnant. *(WSEG = 38/19.0/67.3/8.5)*

SUMMARY

This exercise asked you to practice talking in terms of one doctor treating one patient. Table A3-23 shows the WSEG scores for our revisions.

Table A3-23. **Exercise 5.E. WSEG scores**

	Original				Revision			
	Total words	Avg. words per sentence	Reading ease	Grade level	Total words	Avg. words per sentence	Reading ease	Grade level
	W	S	E	G	W	S	E	G
1	38	38.0	16.8	20.3	37	18.5	60.0	9.4
2	24	24.0	37.9	13.9	23	23	76.8	8.2
3	12	12.0	60.7	7.7	14	14.0	65.7	7.5
4	27	27.0	10.2	18.5	34	17.0	57.7	9.4
5	27	27.0	35.2	15.0	32	16.0	71.6	7.2
6	23	23.0	6.9	18.0	38	19.0	67.3	8.5
Average	25.2	25.2	28.0	15.6	29.7	17.9	66.5	8.4
Change					4.5	−7.3	38.6	−7.2

Chapter 6. Observe the 1066 principle

Exercise 6.A. Prefer the short word to describe the real world

1. Herpes Zoster (HV), caused by the <u>reactivation</u> of latent <u>varicella-zoster</u> virus (VZV) <u>manifests</u> as an acute, painful <u>vesicular</u> rash and is often <u>accompanied</u> by chronic pain or <u>postherpetic</u> <u>neuralgia</u>. *(WSEG = 29/29.0/11.1/18.9)*

Herpes is a real-world problem. Post-herpetic neuralgia is a kind of chronic pain.
  Revision:

> **Herpes Zoster (HV) occurs when a latent <u>varicella-zoster</u> virus (VZV) becomes active. HV shows itself as an acute, painful vesicular rash. The patient may develop <u>post-herpetic neuralgia</u> or other chronic pain.** *(WSEG = 31/10.3/38.0/10.5)*

> **2. Fifth, the airflow <u>limitation</u> or <u>obstruction</u> that happens in COPD is caused by a mixture of small airway disease, <u>parenchymal</u> <u>destruction</u> (<u>emphysema</u>), and, in many cases, increased airways <u>responsiveness</u> (asthma).** *(WSEG = 30/30.0/15.6/18.5)*

This passage talks about real-world lung damage, but the terms, *limitation, obstruction, destruction,* and *responsiveness* sound abstract. We replaced them with the more concrete-sounding terms, *blockage, damage* and *narrowing*.
  Revision:

> **Fifth, the airflow blockage with COPD has a few key causes. They are small airway disease, lung tissue damage (<u>emphysema</u>), and, in many cases, other airway narrowing (asthma).** *(WSEG = 28/14.0/ 56.6/8.8)*

> **3. <u>Maintenance</u> of <u>nocturnal</u> <u>euglycemia</u> is <u>extremely</u> <u>important</u> and is challenging, since most cases of severe <u>hypoglycemia</u> occur at night.** *(WSEG = 19/19.0/4.9/17.2)*

Low blood sugar is a real-world problem. Measuring it is an abstract process.
  Revision:

> **Keeping a patient's nighttime blood sugar level near normal is both important and challenging. Most cases of severe low blood sugar occur at night.** *(WSEG = 24/12.0/60.7/7.7)*

4. <u>Similarly</u>, patients with <u>diabetes</u> had a lower risk of <u>arterial</u> <u>thrombosis</u> than those without <u>diabetes</u>. *(WSEG = 15/15.0/ 22.4/13.8)*

The risk of a blood clot is a real-world problem. Quantifying the risk involves an abstract math calculation.

Revision:

Likewise, a patient who had <u>diabetes</u> had a lower risk of <u>arterial</u> <u>thrombosis</u> than one who did not. *(WSEG = 18/18.0/52.2/10.4)*

5. Immune <u>responses</u> are <u>orchestrated</u> by a complex, <u>continually</u> evolving <u>cooperative</u> network of mobile cells and their products. *(WSEG = 17/17.0/15.4/15.3)*

Immune response is a real-world phenomenon.

Revision:

Immune response involves an ever-changing network of mobile cells and their products that work in concert. *(WSEG = 16/16.0/53.1/9.8)*

6. The initial workup for <u>urticaria</u> and <u>angioedema</u> is a history and <u>physical</u> <u>examination</u> to <u>determine</u> a <u>possible</u> <u>etiology</u>. *(WSEG = 18/ 18.0/0.0/20.2)*

Hives is a synonym for *urticaria. Giant hives* is a synonym for *angioedema*.[1] Hives and giant hives are real-world problems. Getting a history and doing a physical are real-world actions. Medical diagnosis involves abstract thought.

Revision:

The initial workup for hives or giant hives is a history and physical. This data is used to figure out the likely cause. *(WSEG = 23/11.5/ 70.1/6.3)*

SUMMARY

This exercise asked you to practice using short words to describe the real world. Table A3-24 shows the *WSEG* scores for our revisions.

Table A3-24. **Exercise 6.A. WSEG scores**

	Original				Revision			
	Total words	Avg. words per sentence	Reading ease	Grade level	Total words	Avg. words per sentence	Reading ease	Grade level
	W	*S*	*E*	*G*	*W*	*S*	*E*	*G*
1	29	29.0	11.1	18.9	31	10.3	38.0	10.5
2	30	30.0	15.6	18.5	28	14.0	56.6	8.8
3	19	19.0	4.9	17.2	24	12.0	60.7	7.7
4	15	15.0	22.4	13.8	18	18.0	52.2	10.4
5	17	17.0	15.4	15.3	16	16.0	53.1	9.8
6	18	18.0	0.0	20.2	23	11.5	70.1	6.3
Average	21.3	21.3	11.6	17.3	23.3	13.6	55.1	8.9
Change					2.0	−7.7	43.6	−8.4

Exercise 6.B. Prefer's to show real-world possession or connection

1. Within each of these 2 cohorts, we compared the effectiveness of each intervention with a control (sleep hygiene informational video). *(WSEG = 20/20.0/25.7/14.6)*

Cohort and *effectiveness* are abstract concepts. *Intervention* involves real-world activity. *A sleep hygiene informational video* is real-world.

Revision:

Within each cohort, we compared the intervention's effect with a control. The control was a video on sleep hygiene. *(WSEG = 19/9.5/ 59.1/ 7.3)*

2. In this report and the accompanying appendix, we present the data, methods and key findings of the Global Burden of Disease Study 2010 on levels, trends, and age patterns of mortality world-wide. *(WSEG = 32/32.0/28.9/17.1)*

Data, method, finding, level, trend, age pattern and *mortality* are abstract ideas. An appendix is part of the report.

Revision:

> **In this report, we present the data, methods and key findings from the Global Burden of Disease Study 2010. We discuss global death rates, trends, and age patterns.** *(wseg = 28/14.0/59.6/8.4)*

> **3. Importantly, these trials all examine the initiation of therapy with vitamin K antagonists and use as a primary end point the percentage of time that a patient is within the therapeutic range during the initial phase of treatment.** *(wseg = 38/38.0/21.3/19.7)*

This trial involves real-world activity and abstract analysis of the results. Therapeutic range is an abstract idea.

Revision:

> **These trials consider first treatment with a vitamin K antagonist. The main study outcome is how much of the time a patient stays within the therapeutic range during the first treatment phase.** *(wseg = 32/16.0/61.0/8.7)*

> **4. Systematic reviews of diagnostic studies involve additional challenges to those of therapeutic studies.** *(wseg = 13/13.0/0.0/17.6)*

Reading a study is a real-world activity; analyzing it involves abstract thought.

Revision:

> **It is harder to do a systematic review of diagnostic studies than to do one of treatment studies.** *(wseg = 18/18.0/52.2/10.4)*

> **5. Randomized clinical trials are essential to evaluate therapies that reduce rather than eliminate a complication of a disease.** *(wseg = 18/18.0/9.9/16.3)*

A *disease complication* might involve something you can see in the real world. Otherwise, this sounds abstract.

Revision:

> **It takes a randomized clinical trial to test any treatment that reduces a disease complication, but does not cure it.** *(wseg = 20/20.0/51.5/11.0)*

> **6. The U.S. Preventive Services Task Force recommends routine HIV screening, known as opt-out screening, regardless of patient or physician perception of risk for all persons 15 to 65 years of age, unless a patient refuses.** *(wseg = 35/35.0/31.1/17.6)*

The risk of getting HIV is a real-world risk. What people *think* about that risk is abstract.

Revision:

> **The US Preventive Services Task Force recommends routinely screening each patient age 15 to 65 for HIV. This screening should be done without regard for how the doctor or the patient perceive the risk, unless the patient refuses. This is known as "opt-out screening."** (*WSEG* = 44/14.6/63.1/8.0)

SUMMARY

This exercise asked you think about real-world vs. abstract possession or connection. Table A3-25 shows the *WSEG* scores for our revisions.

Table A3-25. **Exercise 6.B.** *WSEG* **scores**

	Original				Revision			
	Total words	Avg. words per sentence	Reading ease	Grade level	Total words	Avg. words per sentence	Reading ease	Grade level
	W	S	E	G	W	S	E	G
1	20	20.0	25.7	14.6	19	9.5	59.1	7.3
2	32	32.0	28.9	17.1	28	14.0	59.6	8.4
3	38	38.0	21.3	19.7	32	16.0	61.0	8.7
4	13	13.0	0.0	17.6	18	18.0	52.2	10.4
5	18	18.0	9.9	16.3	20	20.0	51.5	11.0
6	35	35.0	31.1	17.6	44	14.6	63.1	8.0
Average	26.0	26.0	19.5	17.2	26.8	15.4	57.8	9.0
Change					0.8	−10.7	38.3	−8.2

Exercise 6.C. Use terms consistently; avoid elegant variation

1. **Portenoy states the problem is a <u>lack of studies</u>, not positive results. Even though there is <u>minimal literature</u> on long-term efficacy of opioids for chronic noncancer pain, the <u>few studies</u> that have been published have failed to find good evidence for efficacy.** (*WSEG* = 42/21.0/42.5/12.5)

Revision:

> Portenoy states the problem is a <u>lack of studies</u>, not positive results. True, there are <u>few studies</u> on the long-term effect of opioids to treat chronic non-cancer pain. But <u>those few</u> failed to find good evidence of effectiveness. *(WSEG = 38/12.6/62.6/7.6)*

2. Estimates from WHO's Global Burden of Disease and Risk Factors project show that in 2001, COPD was the fifth leading cause of death in <u>high-income countries</u>, accounting for 3.8% of total deaths, and it was the sixth leading cause of death in <u>nations of low and middle income</u>, accounting for 4.9% of total deaths. *(WSEG = 54/54.0/23.5/23.3)*

Revision:

> In 2001, COPD was the fifth leading cause of death in <u>high-income countries</u>, where it accounted for 3.8% of total deaths. It was also the sixth leading cause of death in <u>low- and middle-income countries</u>, where it accounted for 4.9% of total deaths. (Estimates from WHO's Global Burden of Disease and Risk Factors project.) *(WSEG = 54/18.0/56.9/9.7)*

3. Many legislatures and regulatory boards have adopted model pain <u>statutes</u> that encourage <u>compliance</u> with established <u>standards</u> for prescribing of pharmacologic agents for pain and other symptoms and that protect physicians who <u>observe</u> these <u>guidelines</u> from <u>regulatory intrusion</u> and possible <u>prosecution</u>. *(WSEG = 40/40.0/0.0/25.0)*

In this excerpt, we found three sets of similar terms.
Revision:

> Many legislatures and regulatory boards have adopted model pain <u>laws</u>. These <u>laws</u> encourage a doctor to <u>comply</u> with <u>standards</u> for prescribing a drug to treat pain or other symptoms. They also help shield a doctor who <u>complies</u> from <u>prosecution</u>. *(WSEG = 39/13.0/52.6/9.1)*

4. With the emergence of new direct acting <u>antivirals</u>, the <u>treatment paradigm</u> for <u>hepatitis C virus (HCV) infection</u> is currently undergoing its greatest change since the discovery of <u>the virus</u> 25 years ago. New data are routinely released for different combinations of these new <u>agents</u>, each reporting exceptionally high sustained response rates for an <u>infection</u> that was once notoriously difficult to treat. It is therefore difficult (even for those practicing in the field) to keep abreast of present <u>treatment options</u>, or what is likely to be available in the next 12-18 months. Because newer <u>antivirals</u>

have recently been licensed in the United States and Europe, and the results of several promising large phase III studies have been recently published, now is an opportune time to review the current <u>treatment</u> <u>landscape</u> for <u>HCV</u>, and to anticipate how that <u>landscape</u> might look in coming years. *(WSEG = 142/35.5/24.8/18.6)*

Revision:

New direct acting <u>anti-virals</u> are causing the biggest change in the <u>treatment</u> for <u>hepatitis C virus (HCV)</u> since <u>it</u> was discovered 25 years ago. New data is routinely released for different combinations of these new <u>anti-virals</u>. Each report shows a high sustained response rate. Therefore, it is hard, even for those who practice in the field, to keep abreast of present <u>treatment</u> <u>options</u>. It is also hard to know what will be available in the next year or so.

New <u>anti-virals</u> have lately been licensed in the United States and Europe. The results of several promising large phase III studies have now been published. Therefore, now is a good time to review the current <u>treatment</u> <u>options</u> for <u>HCV</u> and to talk about how those <u>options</u> might look in coming years. *(WSEG = 130/16.2/62.1/8.6)*

5. <u>Men taking zolpidem</u> are at an <u>increased risk of major injury</u>. Compared with the corresponding comparison cohort, <u>the male zolpidem user cohort</u> had a <u>higher risk of major injury</u>. *(WSEG = 29/14.5/40.4/11.2)*

Revision:

<u>Men taking zolpidem</u> had a higher <u>risk of major injury</u> compared to the control group. *(WSEG = 15/15/56.2/9.1)*

6. Celiac disease occurs in persons of European <u>ancestry</u> and in those of Middle Eastern, Indian, South American, and North African <u>descent</u>. It is rare in persons of Asian <u>descent</u>. *(WSEG = 29/14.5/43.3/10.8)*

Revision:

Celiac disease occurs in people of European, Middle Eastern, Indian, South American, or North African <u>descent</u>. It is rare in people of Asian <u>descent</u>. *(WSEG = 24/12.0/39.5/10.7)*

SUMMARY

This exercise asked you to practice using terms consistently. Table A3-26 shows the *WSEG* scores for our revisions.

Table A3-26. **Exercise 6.C. WSEG scores**

	Original				Revision			
	Total words	*Avg. words per sentence*	*Reading ease*	*Grade level*	*Total words*	*Avg. words per sentence*	*Reading ease*	*Grade level*
	W	*S*	*E*	*G*	*W*	*S*	*E*	*G*
1	42	21.0	42.5	12.5	38	12.6	62.6	7.6
2	54	54.0	23.5	23.3	54	18.0	56.9	9.7
3	40	40.0	0.0	25.0	39	13.0	52.6	9.1
4	142	35.5	24.8	18.6	130	16.2	62.1	8.6
5	29	14.5	40.4	11.2	15	15.0	56.2	9.1
6	29	14.5	43.3	10.8	24	12.0	39.5	10.7
Average	56	29.9	29.1	16.9	50.0	14.5	55.0	9.1
Change					−6.0	−15.5	25.9	−7.8

6.D. AVOID USING A LONG, LATIN WORD TO DESCRIBE THE REAL WORLD

1. The risk of HZ is elevated by 1.5 to 2 times in patients with rheumatic and immune-<u>mediated</u> diseases such as rheumatoid arthritis (RA) and Crohn's disease. *(WSEG = 26/26.0/27.5/15.8)*

This sentence talks about a real-world relationship between an immune-related disease and HZ.

Revision:

The risk of HZ is 1.5 to 2 times greater in a patient with an immune-related disease. This would include, e.g., rheumatoid arthritis (RA) or Crohn's disease. *(WSEG = 27/13.5/58.3/8.4)*

2. We hypothesize that rare ADRB2 variants <u>modulate</u> therapeutic responses to LABA therapy and contribute to rare, severe adverse events. *(WSEG = 19/19.0/13.8/16.0)*

This sentence proposes a real-world relationship between rare ADRB2 variants and a patient's response to LABA treatment.

Revision:

We think rare ADRB2 variants may affect a patient's response to LABA treatment. They may also help cause rare but severe adverse events. *(WSEG = 23/11.5/70.1/6.3)*

3. Among the 54 patients, we identified 5 who could willfully <u>modulate</u> their brain activity (Figure 1). *(WSEG = 16/16.0/31.9/12.7)*

This sentence talks about real-world patients who could change their brain activity.
  Revision:

Among the 54 patients, we found 5 could change their brain activity at will (Figure 1). *(WSEG = 16/16.0/68.9/7.6)*

4. Transparency of the <u>regulatory</u> system is also required to overcome several dysfunctions in the drug industry's behaviour. *(WSEG = 17/17.0/0.4/17.4)*

This sentence uses the word *regulatory* in its common, non-medical sense, which is abstract.
  Revision:

We need a regulatory system that is more open. This could help fix some of the drug industry's poor behavior. *(WSEG = 20/10.0/65.5/6.6)*

5. Some experimental support exists for the concept that the ability to discriminate between "self" and "nonself" involves learning to respond aggressively when there are signals that suggest the presence of invasive pathogens and having effective <u>regulatory</u> mechanisms for suppressing inflammatory responses when such signals are absent. *(WSEG = 46/46.0/0.0/26.2)*

The working of the body's immune response is real-world.
  Revision:

To distinguish between "self" and "non-self," the body must learn to respond to a signal that a pathogen is present. It must also have a way to suppress immune response when there is no such signal. Some research supports this idea. *(WSEG = 41/13.6/71.2/6.7)*

6. Urticaria and angioedema are thought to have similar underlying pathophysiological mechanisms, with histamine and other <u>mediators</u> being released from mast cells and basophils. *(WSEG = 23/23.0/0.0/20.0)*

This sentence describes something in the real-world.
  Revision:

Hives and giant hives (*angioedema*) have the same underlying cause. A mast cell or a basophil gives off histamine or other immune response. *(WSEG = 23/11.5/59.0/7.8)*

SUMMARY

This exercise asked you to practice talking about the real world using short, concrete-sounding words. Table A3-27 shows the *WSEG* scores for our revisions.

Table A3-27. **Exercise 6.D. WSEG scores**

	Original				Revision			
	Total words	Avg. words per sentence	Reading ease	Grade level	Total words	Avg. words per sentence	Reading ease	Grade level
	W	*S*	*E*	*G*	*W*	*S*	*E*	*G*
1	26	26.0	27.5	15.8	27	13.5	58.3	8.4
2	19	19.0	13.8	16.0	23	11.5	70.1	6.3
3	16	16.0	31.9	12.7	16	16.0	68.9	7.6
4	17	17.0	0.4	17.4	20	10.0	65.5	6.6
5	46	46.0	0.0	26.2	41	13.6	71.2	6.7
6	23	23.0	0.0	20.0	23	11.5	59.0	7.8
Average	24.5	24.5	12.3	18.0	25.0	12.7	65.5	7.2
Change					0.5	−11.8	53.2	−10.8

Chapter 7. Statistical analysis of WSEG scores

Exercise 7. Putting the tips on reading ease and vivid language into practice
Here are some of the symptoms we observed:

- Long sentence: One sentence is 39 words long, another is 36 words long. The average sentence length (24.8 words) seems high.
- Run-on sentence: The 39-word sentence seems to cover two ideas. We would split it into two.
- Dependent clause: The 36-word sentence starts with a long dependent clause. This pushes the subject and verb away from the start of the sentence.
- Long words: There are many long words, but only a few essential scientific terms. In our revision, we only used *intensive care unit (ICU), therapeutic trial, palliative care,* and *cross-sectional study.* This paragraph has a high percentage of long words (28/149 = 19%). This seems high for an excerpt with low science content.

- Elegant variation: (a) *critical care specialists, ICU physicians, ICU clinicians, health care providers;* (b) *an acceptable health state for the patient, an outcome that patients can meaningfully appreciate;* (c) *critical care, intensive care, aggressive critical care, intensive care interventions, care, therapeutic, treatment;* and (d) *specialists, physicians, clinicians, health care providers.*
- Passive voice: *should be considered, are often perceived.*
- Abstract language: The many long words tend to sound abstract. The narrative uses many plural subjects and objects, which tend to sound more abstract than those in the singular.
- Formality: The long words also tend to sound formal.
- Nominalization: *admission, transition, interventions, providers.*

Revision:

> **When a doctor treats a patient in an intensive care unit (ICU), they can either save a life or give futile care that just delays death. Therefore, a doctor should think of putting a patient in an ICU as a therapeutic trial. Once the doctor sees the patient will never recover, they should send them to palliative care.**
>
> **Sadly, ICU doctors sometimes give a patient futile care. A survey of Canadian ICU doctors found 87% believed their ICU had given some futile care in the past year. A one-day cross-sectional study performed in Europe found 27% of ICU doctors believed they gave at least 1 patient "inappropriate" care. What made it so? The most common answer: it was too much.** *(WSEG = 120/15.0/61.8/8.3)*

Chapter 8. Organize your narrative in a way that's helpful for your reader

Exercise 8.A. Introduce and develop a single idea in each paragraph
1. We find this paragraph challenging and we feel we need to study it. We think it covers multiple ideas.

Revision:

> *What happens during metabolism?*
>
> **In a majority of cases, metabolism that is mediated by cytochrome P-450 represents a deactivation pathway. For some drugs, however, oxidation leads to conversion of a prodrug into an active compound. (31 words)**

What are some examples of a CYP- gene activating a pro-drug?

A prime example is codeine (metabolized by CYP2D6); other examples include clopidogrel (metabolized by CYP3A4), cyclophosphamide (metabolized by CYP2B6) and tamoxifen (metabolized by CYP2D6). (24 words)

What are the metabolic processes CYP2D6 triggers in codeine?

The major pathway of codeine consists of glucuronidation and N-demethylation, whereas the CYP2D6-mediated O-demethylation to produce morphine is a minor reaction. Nevertheless, the latter is a crucial step in bioactivation, since the affinity of codeine for the μ-opioid receptor is only 1/200 to 1/3000 that of morphine. (47 words)

How does genetic variation effect how a patient metabolizes codeine?

Previous studies have shown that the effects of codeine—analgesic, respiratory, psychomotor, and miotic—are markedly attenuated in people with poor metabolism of CYP2D6. On the other hand, people with ultrarapid metabolism, such as the patient described by Gasche et al. in this issue of the *Journal*, produce greater amounts of morphine from codeine and therefore may experience exaggerated pharmacologic effects in response to regular doses of codeine. (68 words)

How does genetic variation effect how a patient metabolizes other drugs?

Similar effects, albeit less dramatic, have been described in patients with ultrarapid metabolism of CYP2D6 in response to routine doses of hydrocodone or oxycodone, which are other opioids requiring CYP2D6 mediated activation. These reports clearly illustrate the effect of CYP2D6 genetic polymorphisms on the action of codeine, ranging from virtually no effect in patients with poor metabolism to severe toxic effects in those with ultrarapid metabolism. (66 words)

How common is it for a patient to have a genetic variation that effects how they metabolize a drug?

To put these observations into perspective, these extremes of response might be relevant for some 10 to 20 percent of whites who have phenotypes associated with either poor metabolism or ultra-rapid metabolism. (32 words)

We think the shorter paragraphs and headings help a reader to scan the article and get the "big picture" quickly before reading the details.

2. We feel we need to study this paragraph. We think this paragraph covers multiple ideas.

Revision:

Pulmonary Artery Catheter (PAC)—The clinical gold standard for estimating CO

The [pulmonary artery catheter] PAC, today still considered the clinical gold standard for CO estimation, gives three fundamental bits of hemodynamic information: CO, pulmonary and cardiac filling pressures and mixed SvO_2. The PAC is considered the clinical gold standard or reference method for CO estimation and every new tool built for CO estimation has to be compared with PAC in validation studies. (59 words)

How can you use the PAC to measure macro circulation?

The technique is based on the injection of an ice-cold solution into the right atrium (proximal port—prox injectate—blue lumen). The change in blood temperature is measured in the pulmonary artery by a thermistor placed proximally to the tip of the catheter. The thermo dilution curve is used for CO estimation by means of the Steward-Hamilton formulation. The measurement is repeated at least three to five times (in order to compensate for variations induced by the respiratory cycle) and the average value is then calculated. (86 words)

How can you use a PAC to obtain an inverted thermodilution curve?

An "inverted" thermodilution curve can be obtained by worming [sic] the blood with a thermal filament (Vigilance™, Edwards Lifesciences, Irvine, CA, USA) or a thermal coil (OptiQ™, ICU Medical, San Clemente, CA, USA). This system allows for a semi-continuous CO measurement by displaying average CO Values for the previous 10 min and limiting, for this reason, the effects of arrhythmias and other compounding factors. Although the CO value is frequently updated, this type of monitoring is not continuous (beat-by-beat) and is therefore less accurate and rapid in detecting hemodynamic instability. (89 words)

What are limiting factors for estimating CO?

Major limiting factors for CO estimation with any type of thermodilution is the occurrence of tricuspid regurgitation and intracardiac shunts. In fact, prolonged indicator transit times or indicator recycling may lead to errors in CO estimation. SvO_2 suggests whether or not cardiac output is adequate in a patient since it provides a useful indication about the adequacy of tissue oxygenation in specific conditions of metabolic activity. When SvO_2 decreases below normal values (70–75%) in the presence of normal arterial oxygen saturation and without anemia, it means that CO is inadequate and measures aimed at increasing DO_2 should be promptly implemented. (100 words)

What are the different ways to measure SvO₂?

SvO_2 can be measured either continuously (fiberoptic fibers) or intermittently by withdrawing a mixed venous blood sample from the distal lumen of the PAC. The PAC measures: the pulmonary artery pressure which represents right ventricular afterload; right atrial pressure (RAP/CVP, PAOP) have been demonstrated to be less reliable than dynamic indicators of fluid responsiveness (pulse pressure variations PPV, systolic pressure variation SPV and stroke volume variation SVV). Nonetheless, when static parameters are particularly low, they can be considered to be as reliable as dynamic ones. (86 words)

What is the recent trend in using PAC?

Over recent years, the use of PAC has decreased significantly for two main reasons: firstly, several randomized and non-randomized studies have not demonstrated an improvement in patient outcomes when therapies were guided by PAC and secondly nowadays the PAC is the most invasive tool for hemodynamic monitoring currently used in ICUs or ORs. In 1996, Connors and co-workers published in *JAMA* a prospective cohort study in which the authors used case-matching multivariable regression modeling techniques and a propensity score. The results showed that pulmonary artery catheterization in critically ill patients was associated with an increased risk of death (odds ratio 1.24; 95% confidence interval 1.03–1.49) as well as a prolonged length of stay and increased resource utilization. (117 words)

What was the aftermath of the Connors and co-workers study?

After this shocking paper, a litany of randomized trials aimed at confirming these results was performed in ICUs. The net results of this great amount of data corresponded to an increased suspicion that PAC-guided treatment may not be superior to non-PAC-guided treatment and a marked decrease in PAC use worldwide has become clear during the last 10–15 years. In the USA, Wiener et al. reported a 65% decrease in PAC use between 1993 and 2004 and in Canada, Koo et al. reported a more than 50% decrease between 2002 and 2006. A great number of papers has been published by opinion leaders and general considerations about the use of PAC and its benefits. (113 words)

What are the doubts about the usefulness of PAC?

The doubts regarding its usefulness can be listed as follows. (10 words)

We think the shorter paragraphs and headings help make the content easier to grasp.

Exercise 8.B. Present two-dimensional data in a table, chart or graph

1. All 525 study participants, who were randomized to receive varenicline or placebo, had been diagnosed with major depressive disorder and were being treated with antidepressant drugs at a stable dose or had been successfully treated for depression within the past 2 years. <u>At 9 to 12 weeks, 35.9% of those who received varenicline quit vs 15.6% taking placebo; at 40 weeks, 20.3% of the varenicline group had quit compared with 10.4% of the placebo group.</u> Depression and anxiety did not increase in either group, but the researchers cautioned that their findings may not apply to smokers whose depression isn't successfully treated. *(WSEG = 101/33.6/30.4/15.2)*

Revision:

Each of the 525 study participants was chosen at random to receive varenicline or placebo. Each had been diagnosed with major depressive disorder. Each was being treated with antidepressant drugs at a stable dose or had been treated for depression, with success, within the past 2 years. Table A3-28 shows the results.

Table A3-28. **Study subjects who quit smoking**

	Received varenicline	*Received placebo*
At 9 to 12 weeks	35.9%	15.6%
At 40 weeks	20.3%	10.4%

Depression and anxiety did not increase in either group. But the researchers cautioned, their findings might not apply to a smoker whose depression is not treated with success. *(WSEG = 80/13.5/55.8/ 8.7, excludes table)*

2. What about health in Scotland? According to the UK's national statistical office, <u>healthy life expectancy was 59·8 years for men and 64·1 years for women</u> in Scotland during 2008–10, <u>4·6 years and 2·3 years fewer than for men and women in England, respectively</u>. According to the British Heart Foundation, <u>35% of Scottish men and 30% of women have high blood pressure;</u> alcohol use is one noticeable contributor to ill health in Scotland, with up to <u>50% of</u>

men and 30% of women exceeding guidelines for drinking. *(WSEG = 87/29.0/37.9/13.3)*

Revision:

What about health in Scotland? (Table A3-29)

Table A3-29. **Some key data on health in Scotland**

	Men	*Women*
Healthy life expectancy (years)[1]	59.8	64.1
Difference compared to England (years)[1]	(4.6)	(2.3)
High blood pressure[2]	35%	30%
Alcohol use exceeding guidelines[2]	50%	30%

Sources:
1. UK national statistical office; data for 2008–10
2. British Heart Foundation

Alcohol use is one noticeable contributor to ill health in Scotland.

(WSEG = 18/8.0/55.9/7.4, excludes table)
You might instead present the data in the form of a chart or graph. Figures A3-1 and A3-2.

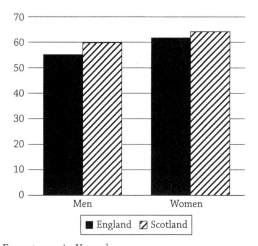

Figure A3-1 Life Expectancy in Years.[1]

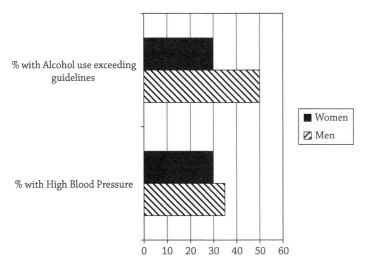

Figure A3-2 Scotland Health.[2]
Sources: 1. UK national statistical office; data for 2008–10
2. British Heart Foundation.

Chapter 9. Choose a clear narrative pathway

Exercise 9.A. Start with things known
We don't think the excerpt starts by talking about concepts familiar to the widest reasonable audience. It starts by reviewing kidney anatomy, which an engineer or a mathematician might not know.

Exercise 9.B. Start by anchoring the discussion in the real world
You might say the narrative starts by talking about the real world since a kidney is something in the real world. But "mammal" is the name for an abstract biological class. Likewise, the concept of a "mammal kidney" is an abstract idea. It assumes kidneys from different mammals are enough alike that it makes sense to generalize.

Exercise 9.C. Choose a good narrative pathway
1. We see three narrative pathways: (a) kidney anatomy—big to small, (b) rat kidney vs. human kidney, and (c) blood flow—upstream to downstream.
2. The narrative doesn't state them explicitly, but they are clear from context.
3. The narrative doesn't follow them consistently. We saw some issues that interrupt the narrative flow:
   - The narrative of "kidney anatomy—big to small" changes direction at one point and goes from smaller to bigger (inner medulla + outer medulla = medulla).

- The big-to-small narrative also gets interrupted by comparing a rat kidney to a human kidney.
- There is a gap in the big-to-small narrative. It never explains where a nephron belongs in relation to the large parts of the kidney: cortex, inner medulla, and outer medulla.

Exercise 9.D. Make a smooth transition between concrete and abstract

1. The real world objects the narrative mentions are cortex, inner and outer medulla, nephron, rat kidney, human kidney, renal corpuscle, renal tubule, glomerulus, Bowman's capsule, capillaries, arterioles, water and blood. The main real world action is blood flow.

    The concept of a mammal is an abstract biological classification. Likewise, the generalized concept of a mammal kidney is abstract. The ideas, "specialized for absorption and secretion," and "pressure gradient" also sound abstract.

    It might be possible to revise the discussion of real-world blood flow to use more concrete-sounding terms (e.g., soaks up or absorbs rather than absorption; and empties into, gives off, or secretes rather than secretion.) It might also make for a smoother transition to keep real-world anatomy, real-world blood flow, and abstract ideas in separate sentences or paragraphs.

2. Both a rat kidney and a human kidney are made up of bundles of tiny nephrons that filter blood. The size and shape of an individual nephron are similar. The main difference is, a human kidney is bigger because it has many more nephrons. The narrative doesn't mention this.

3. All mammal kidneys consist of bundles of tiny nephrons. As the size of the mammal increases, the size and shape of an individual nephron stays about the same, but the number of nephrons increases. The narrative also doesn't mention this.

4. All mammal kidneys are enough alike that it makes sense to generalize about a typical mammal kidney. A kidney, whether of a rat, a human, an elephant or a whale, is composed of bundles of tiny nephrons that filter wastes and toxins out of the blood and channels them to make urine. The size and shape of an individual nephron is similar for any mammal. Bigger mammals have more nephrons: a rat kidney has about 38,000 nephrons. A human kidney has about 1 million nephrons.

Chapter 10. Forge a strong chain of logical reasoning

Exercise 10.A. Explain each step of reasoning

1. A nephron is located partly in the cortex and partly in the medulla.

2. The narrative doesn't explain this. Therefore, it appears to have left out a step of reasoning. (The article does show this later in a figure.)

Exercise 10.B. State the problem before you solve it
1. If a patient's kidney stops filtering blood, they will die unless they receive dialysis.
2. A math model of how the kidney filters blood might help design a dialysis machine that better mimics kidney function. It might also lead to better treatment or prevention of kidney disease.
3. There is no statement of the problem math modeling helps solve in this excerpt. (But the article does mention this elsewhere.)

Exercise 10.C. Say it in words before you say it in symbols
1. The narrative explains the three equations in general terms but doesn't explain each individual equation. We found the narrative confusing. We would like to see the equations explained more clearly. For example, the narrative describes the three equations as *ODE's* (ordinary differential equations?) but uses the notation for partial derivatives (δ_x). We also found the explanation of variables unclear (e.g., what does C_{pr} stand for?)
2. The widest reasonable audience probably needs: (1) for those who have forgotten calculus, a brief summary of the model; and (2) for those who haven't forgotten calculus, a careful, step-by-step tour.

Note

1. *Stedman's Medical Dictionary*, s.vv. "Urticaria," "Angioedema."

GLOSSARY

The 1066 Principle—the general tendency for English speakers to use short words to talk about the real world, and long words, more sparingly, to talk about abstract ideas.

Abstract—a theoretical way of looking at things; something that exists only in idealized form. A term is abstract if it relates to the world of ideas, including a concept, theory, calculation or procedure. Contrast with *concrete.*

Active voice—A sentence is in active voice when its subject is *doing* the action. See *voice.*

Clear—Writing is *clear* when the narrative uses words and concepts familiar to the reader. Ideally, a reader can understand and vividly imagine the article on first reading without having to *study* it. The reader remembers each key idea.

Closed compound—a compound word written as one word (e.g., *multicell, hyperadrenergic, vasomotor,* and *sinoatrial).* See *compound word.*

Compound word or *compound*—a word formed by combining two or more words, or a word plus a prefix. The three main types of compounds are the *open compound* (e.g., *student nurse),* the *closed compound* (e.g., *multicell),* and the *hyphenated compound* (e.g., *pre-menstrual).*

Concise—Writing is *concise* when it demands as little of the reader's mental energy as possible. This usually means short while still clear. Good writing involves tradeoffs. A few short words may convey the message more vividly than one long, but lifeless word. Writing concisely often means cutting any unnecessary word; but sometimes, cutting too many words makes the message cryptic and harder to understand.

Concrete—something from the real world (e.g., a doctor, a patient, a bed, a test tube). Contrast with *abstract.*

Elegant variation—varying terms to make writing more interesting. Technical writing tends to avoid elegant variation, but it is common in other types of writing.

Essential scientific content—important scientific ideas an author must include in their article.

Essential scientific term—a long word that helps convey essential scientific content clearly and concisely. An essential scientific term meets four tests:

1. No shorter word serves just as well,
2. You can't paraphrase in a few short words,
3. Doctors and other medical scientists use the term consistently (i.e., exclusively), and
4. It's easy to look up in a standard reference.

False signal—using an abstract-sounding word to talk about something in the real world, or a concrete-sounding word to talk about something abstract. Contrast with *signal.*

Flesch Reading Ease—a readability test that indicates how difficult it is to read a passage in English. The scores generally range from 0.0 to 100.0.

Flesch-Kincaid Grade Level—a readability test that assigns a USA school grade level or year to a passage in English.

Hyphenated compound—a compound word where words are written together but separated by a hyphen (e.g., *pre-menstrual, cost-effective, one-time, self-reported*). See *compound word*.

Insider—somebody who knows the science and vocabulary of a particular specialized field. *Insiders* are the narrowest possible definition of the potential audience for an article. Contrast with the *widest reasonable audience*.

Long word—any word with three or more syllables, but not including a two-syllable word that becomes a three-syllable word by adding a common ending, such as *-ed, -es* or *-ing*.

Medicus incomprehensibilis—a condition that affects doctors and other medical scientists and causes them to write dull, lifeless prose that is hard to understand. *Medicus incomprehensibilis* is primarily caused by needless grammatical complexity.

Narrative pathway—the direction of a narrative, or a conceptual program for organizing a narrative.

Nominalization—the process of making an abstract noun out of a verb or adjective.

Noun string—a group of nouns and their modifiers. Often, a noun string consists of obscure technical terms. Multiple terms may function together as an adjective.

Open compound—a compound word, where words work together, but are written as separate words (e.g., *student nurse, 50 percent, reference book*). See *compound word*.

Passive voice—A sentence is in passive voice when its subject receives the action. See *voice*.

Past participle—a form of the verb that expresses completed action.[1] A past participle is usually the same form as the verb in past tense. For regular verbs, this means adding a *-d* or *-ed* ending (e.g., *worked, decided, starved*). Irregular verbs use irregular forms (e.g., *broken, swum*).[2] Examples:

- "The results of the meta-analysis of treatment effect of lubiprostone vs. placebo are <u>shown</u> in Figures 2 and 3."[3] In this sentence, *shown* is a past participle.
- "It may be <u>specified</u> in the protocol of a prospective accuracy study, for instance, that to reduce study costs or burden to patients only a randomly <u>selected</u> subset of patients in a specific subgroup are to be <u>verified</u> by the <u>preferred</u> reference standard."[4] In this sentence, *specified, selected, verified*, and *preferred* are past participles.

Plain English—writing that conveys the right content, clearly and concisely. Writing in plain English involves sharpening up the medical science to make it clearer and more accessible to the widest reasonable audience.

Short word—a one- or two-syllable word. This also includes a two-syllable word that becomes a three-syllable word by adding a common ending, such as *-ed, -es*, or *-ing*. Contrast with *long word*.

Signal—a way of indicating, through word choice, whether you're talking about the real world or the world of abstract ideas. Short words tend to signal *real world*, and longer words *abstract*. Contrast with *false signal*.

Subject (grammar)—the noun or pronoun that agrees with the verb.[5] A noun functioning as a subject is the actor, person, or thing about which an assertion is made in a clause.[6] Examples:

- "<u>Onychomycosis</u> is a fungal infection of the nails that causes discoloration, thickening, and separation from the nail bed."[7] In this sentence, *Onychomycosis* is the subject.
- "<u>Identification</u> of hyphae, pseudohyphae, or spores confirms infection but does not identify the organism."[8] Here, *Identification* is the subject. (The phrase, *"Identification of hyphae, pseudohyphae, or spores,"* is the *logical* subject.[9])

Verb—expresses an action, occurrence or a state of being.[10] Examples:

- "Diagnostic studies typically <u>evaluate</u> the accuracy of one or more tests, markers, or models by comparing their results with those of, ideally, a "gold" reference test or standard."[11] Here, the verb is *evaluate*.
- "High K⁺ intake also <u>has</u> a stimulatory effect on the release of aldosterone at the level of the adrenal gland."[12] Here, the verb is *has*.

Vivid language—language that is clear, detailed, powerful, full of life, and strikingly alive.

Voice—a term that describes whether the subject of the sentence is doing or receiving the action. See *active voice; passive voice.*

Widest reasonable audience—the widest reasonable audience for a journal article includes anybody with an interest in the science, whether or not they are an *insider* in the field. It includes a doctor or scientist working in the same specialty, another specialty, or even another discipline. It includes someone living or educated in an English-speaking country or elsewhere, whether they are a native speaker of English or not. It includes readers at different levels of training. It includes a regular journal subscriber and somebody who searches for an article on the internet. Contrast with *insider*.

WSEG—four items of data helpful for assessing reading ease for a writing sample: the number of <u>w</u>ords *(w)*, average <u>s</u>entence length *(s)*, Flesch Reading <u>E</u>ase score *(e)*, and Flesch-Kincaid <u>G</u>rade Level *(g)*. We write a *WSEG score* for a writing sample in the form *(WSEG = 55/55.0/0.2/26.8)*.

Notes

1. *Chicago Manual of Style*, 15th ed. §5.103.
2. Williams, *Style: Lessons in Clarity*, 266 (see Preface, n. 8).
3. Li F, et al. "Lubiprostone is Effective in the Treatment of Chronic Idiopathic Constipation and Irritable Bowel Syndrome: A Systematic Review and Meta-Analysis of Randomized Controlled Trials," *Mayo Clinic Proc* 91, no. 4 (2016): 461.
4. Naaktgeboren C, et al. "Anticipating Missing Reference Standard Data When Planning Diagnostic Accuracy Studies," *BMJ* 352 (2016), under "The problem: missing reference standard data," http://www.ncbi.nlm.nih.gov/pmc/articles/PMC4772780/.
5. Cutts, *Oxford Guide to Plain English*, 122 (see chap. 1, n. 6).
6. *The Chicago Manual of Style*, 15th ed. §5.23.
7. Westerberg D, Voyack M, "Onychomycosis: Current Trends in Diagnosis and Treatment," *Am Fam Phys* 88, no. 11 (2013): 762.
8. Ibid.
9. See Williams, *Style: Lessons in Clarity*, 81–82 (see Preface, n. 8).
10. *Merriam-Webster's Learner's Dictionary*, Merriam-Webster.com, (accessed July 11, 2016), http://www.merriam-webster.com/dictionary/verb. s.v. "Verb."
11. Naaktgeboren et al. "Anticipating Missing Reference Standard," (*see Glossary*, n. 4).
12. Palmer B, Clegg D, "Achieving the Benefits of High-Potassium, Paleolithic Diet, Without the Toxicity," *Mayo Clinic Proc* 91, no. 4 (2016): 500.

RESOURCES

Books

Booth, Wayne C., Gregory G. Colomb, Joseph M. Williams. *The Craft of Research*. 3rd ed. Chicago: University of Chicago Press, 2008.

Cutts, Martin. *Oxford Guide to Plain English*. Oxford: Oxford University Press, 2009.

Garner, Bryan A. *The Elements of Legal Style*. 2nd ed. Oxford: Oxford University Press, 2002.

Garner, Bryan A. *Legal Writing in Plain English*. Chicago: University of Chicago Press, 2001.

Garner, Bryan A. *Securities Disclosure in Plain English*. Chicago: CCH Incorporated, 1999.

Greene, Anne E. *Writing Science in Plain English*. Chicago: University of Chicago Press, 2013.

Iverson, Cheryl, et al. *AMA Manual of Style*. 10th ed. Oxford: Oxford University Press, 2007.

Kimble, Joseph. *Lifting the Fog of Legalese*. Durham, NC: Carolina Academic Press, 2006.

Office of Investor Education and Assistance. *A Plain English Handbook*. Washington, DC: US Securities and Exchange Commission, 1998.

Strunk, William, Jr. and E. B. White. *The Elements of Style*. 3rd ed. New York: Macmillan, 1979.

Stedman's Medical Dictionary. 28th ed. Philadelphia: Lippincott Williams & Wilkins, 2006.

Tufte, Edward R. *The Visual Display of Quantitative Information*. 2nd ed. Cheshire, CT: Graphics Press, 2001.

University of Chicago Press. *Chicago Manual of Style*. 15th ed. Chicago: University of Chicago Press, 2003.

Williams, Joseph M. *Style: Lessons in Clarity and Grace*. 9th ed. New York: Pearson Longman, 2007.

Wydick, Richard C. *Plain English for Lawyers*. Durham, NC: Carolina Academic, 2005.

Articles

Gopen, George D., and Judith A. Swan. "The Science of Scientific Writing." *American Scientist* 78 (November–December 1990), http://www.americanscientist.org/issues/pub/the-science-of-scientific-writing/1.

Orwell, George. "Politics and the English Language," *Horizon* (April 1946). Available online, http://www.orwell.ru/library/essays/politics/english/e_polit/.

Internet References

Plain Language Action and Information Network. *Federal Plain Language Guidelines*. (March 2011, revised May 2011), www.plainlanguage.gov.

Plain Language at NIH, National Institutes of Health, https://www.nih.gov/institutes-nih/nih-office-director/office-communications-public-liaison/clear-communication/plain-language.

INDEX

References to figures and tables are denoted by an italicized *f* and *t*